1992

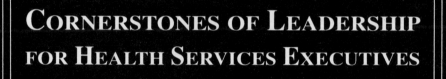

CORNERSTONES OF LEADERSHIP
FOR HEALTH SERVICES EXECUTIVES

AMERICAN COLLEGE OF HEALTHCARE EXECUTIVES MANAGEMENT SERIES

Anthony R. Kovner, Series Editor

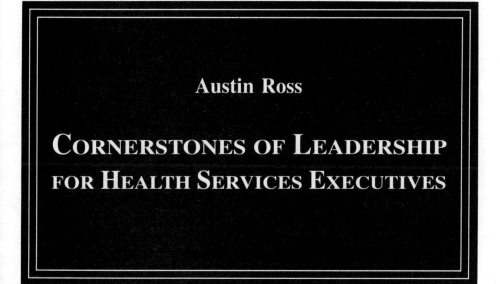

Austin Ross

CORNERSTONES OF LEADERSHIP
FOR HEALTH SERVICES EXECUTIVES

MANAGEMENT SERIES
American College of Healthcare Executives

95 94 93 92 91   5 4 3 2 1

Library of Congress Cataloging-in-Publication Data

Ross, Austin.
   Cornerstones of leadership for health services executives / Austin Ross.
       p.   cm. — (Management series / American College of Healthcare
   Executives)
   Includes bibliographical references and index.
   ISBN 0-910701-58-X (hardbound : alk. paper)
   1. Health services administration.   2. Leadership.   I. Title   II. Series:
   Management series (Ann Arbor, Mich.)
       [DNLM: 1. Health Facility Administrators.   2. Leadership.   WX 155
   R823c]
   RA971.R63   1992   362.1'068'4—dc20
   DNLM/DLC for Library of Congress   91-35345 CIP

The paper used in this publication meets the minimum requirements of American National Standard for Information Sciences—Permanence of Paper for Printed Library Materials, ANSI Z39.48-1984.   ∞™

Health Administration Press
A division of the Foundation of the
   American College of Healthcare Executives
1021 East Huron Street
Ann Arbor, Michigan 48104-9990
(313) 764-1380

For Annette, Carol, Randall, Becky, and Austin T.

CONTENTS

Part III Flexibility: Adapting to Turbulent Times

Part IV Vision: Looking Back and Thinking Ahead

FOREWORD

Austin Ross begins the introduction to this book on leadership by stating that "the essence of leadership is elusive." It is important for readers to know that Austin Ross, in his successful career, has learned what leadership is and has practiced it. He has been recognized as a leader not only in his own organization and community but throughout the nation as well. His 36-year career at the Virginia Mason Medical Center and his national elected leadership positions collectively reflect his unique and capable leadership. Both the American College of Healthcare Executives and the Medical Group Management Association have elevated him to their highest elective office. He has accomplished that of which he now writes.

"The essence of leadership is elusive." It is, at once, a clear and challenging statement. Clear, because there is no misunderstanding: Leadership defies definition. Challenging, because we still must seek to define it. Will I know leadership when I see it? How really elusive is it? Can other people see it although I cannot? If you want a debate on the issue of leadership, just try to get a group consensus in response to the question, "Who were the best leaders among the U.S. presidents in the twentieth century?" Individual conclusions will be reached on the basis of each president's political party, specific success with our national economy, establishment of social programs, and many other parameters. The same would be true in trying to identify our most successful industrial leaders. Should we examine process or outcome? Do individuals really lead or just flow with external forces? Do leaders make the times or do the times make the leaders? It may be that just keeping a company alive is the mark of a leader. On the other hand, maybe true leadership in health care is marked by the ability to close a hospital.

These questions and comments convey the elusive nature of leadership. But in spite of the inherent challenge, attempting to define leadership is a necessary journey, and Austin Ross is a worthy travel guide. Ross's approach to the subject is easy to follow. The text is divided into sections on balance, direction, flexibility, and vision, giving the reader a focus plus insight into Ross's thinking about leadership. Leadership is not all vision; it is a combination of characteristics that change with time. The journey will be exciting.

Health care leadership is a timely issue. Problems and pressures exist everywhere in the system. Employers, elected and appointed government officials, national and local health associations, and just about all of us are involved in discussions about health care. Proposals for "solving the health care crisis" abound, and it appears that we have entered a permanent state of turmoil. If there was ever a time for leadership, it is now. Health care executives have the opportunity to successfully respond to this leadership challenge.

The opportunity for executive leadership in health care has never been this obvious and available. The 1990s and the need to prepare for the twenty-first century provide exciting and limitless leadership opportunities. Major change requires enlightened leadership. The pressure is on. Health care executives must respond.

Do we have enough leaders in health care to face the growing problems? My personal view is that we do not. The reason for the shortage is that health care executives, for the most part, have not had to take the lead in creating change in health care. Government, in particular, has been the major force in setting the overall direction of our health care system. The Hill-Burton Act (1946), the expansion of health-related education and research (1950s–1970s), the establishment of Medicare and Medicaid (1965), and the implementation of the prospective payment system (1983) have all been major contributors to health care change. Along with the movement to managed care and the need for cost-containment strategies, these changes have allowed health care executives to "go with the flow" for the most part. In general, success has been defined as responding well to the changing incentives. Even so, some health care executives have been able to find opportunities for leadership and have moved their organizations in unexpected and rewarding directions.

It is my belief that far more opportunities for leadership will develop in the foreseeable future. Governmental bodies (federal and state) will not be able to provide a detailed blueprint or set of new initiatives to lead us into the future. This conclusion is based upon the significant limitations being placed upon government "solutions" to health care problems because of financial constraints. Clearly, budget deficits do not bode well for creative solutions to health care problems. We have rediscovered that "health is a local affair," and more than ever, health care executives will find opportunities for leadership at their local level. The only question is: Are we ready to respond? Will we know how to respond?

Health care executives must spend more time preparing for leadership roles. They must commit themselves to aggressive programs of learning. This means reading, attending seminars, and taking advantage of other forms of continuing education. It means learning how to speak out in a wide variety of forums, informing people and molding opinion. This cannot be done from one's office or hospital. It must be accomplished in the public forum. The leader must put himself or herself at risk. The leader must spend more time in the community, listening and learning about its problems. Then and only then can the leader take the necessary steps toward creating new approaches or even new organizations to improve the community's health.

The path toward leadership is not clear. But with guidance from Ross and other authors, the trip can begin. Sound advice from "those who have been there" provides an important foundation.

Now, as you move through the four parts of the book—balance, direction, flexibility, and vision—remember that the titles of the parts themselves deliver a basic message. Leadership is many things. But it is, more importantly, a combination of many things. Each part, while described discretely, loses itself in the whole. The reader will be challenged to constantly integrate the words, the chapters, and the four parts. The author has done his part, the reader must now take over.

A final note: Ross emphasizes team building. This is a long-term approach that requires a great commitment on the part of the leader, and it may be one of the secrets to successful leadership. Commitment to staff and effective service as a mentor are the leader's investments in the organization's future. Although team building has been addressed in the literature, Ross concentrates upon a subtle and often neglected aspect of the management-staff relationship: that shift in attitude that turns boss into mentor, employer into teacher, manager into leader.

The importance of team building cannot be overemphasized. Ross sees it as an integral part of the leadership role. So do I. If we leave no one behind to assume our role, we have failed as leaders. Let us understand that our job does not end with today's successes. Tomorrow's success, when we are gone, is a responsibility we hold today. May health care leaders create the vision and the team that can leap beyond the limits of today.

Stuart A. Wesbury, Jr.
President (1979–1991)
American College of Healthcare Executives

PREFACE

This book presents a personal perspective on some of the complicated aspects of directing a complex health care organization. It does not present data or solutions formulated through documented research. Rather, conclusions are based on observations and reflections either made firsthand or assimilated through many contacts with professional colleagues in the hospital and group practice fields.

One of the basic themes in this book is that there are few simple solutions to the problems encountered along the trail to successful leadership. And there are no shortcuts. An individual's leadership style is based on personality, experiments with what works and what doesn't work, and knowledge gained through academics. Management skills and techniques are developed throughout one's career with the application of energy and concentration. However, the leader's success is dependent on the ability to put all of these skills into practice, and this is the artistic side of leading that is so difficult to define.

As industries experience the kind of rapid change that is now most characteristic of health services, excellence in leadership is both absolutely essential and harder to achieve. Leadership very often determines whether an organization grows, prospers, and is socially productive or is stagnant and unable to survive the rapid pace of change. This book focuses on leadership practices and principles that are of particular interest and importance to health services executives.

No two of us are exactly alike, so what works for me might not work for you. Readers should test the material in this book by challenging concepts and comparing their own observations with mine. My hope in putting these observations together in a book is that the written word will help readers connect and define their own thoughts and perspectives on leadership. If the reader picks out of these pages even two or three thoughts that are new or reshaped, I will consider the writing assignment successful.

ACKNOWLEDGMENTS

This book could not have been written without the incredible support of my spouse, Annette, who tolerated my off-hours addiction to the process of trying to make sense out of the subtleties of the subject matter.

I am also deeply indebted to Fran Sargent and Patty Carlson, who were so patient with me and helped pull the pieces of the manuscript together.

In addition, the whole project would have floundered if not for Daphne Grew, Director of Health Administration Press, and Sandra Crump, Editor at Health Administration Press. Daphne and Sandra understood from the beginning that executives who embark on complex writing assignments need lots of help and encouragement.

Finally, I am grateful to many colleagues, particularly Don Olson, Bob Boyle, Mike Rona, Roger Lindeman, Mark Secord, Joyce Jackson, and Ned Borgstrom, who not only provided lots of advice but also assisted, perhaps inadvertently at times, by participating in a "living laboratory" on leadership issues.

INTRODUCTION

THE CHALLENGE TO CONTEMPORARY LEADERS IN HEALTH CARE

Leadership is one of the most observed and least understood phenomena on earth.

James McGregor Burns, *Leadership*

Describing excellence in health care leadership is a little like the parable of the six blind men who tried to describe an elephant: one by touching the trunk, the second the tail, the third the hide, and so forth. Try as we might to define it, in many ways the essence of leadership is elusive. The leader's success depends on so many variables—the environment and culture of the organization, the talent the leader brings to the organization, the quality of the leader's past experiences—that no formula for success can be prescribed. No two people experience or view their role in the same way, and each brings a different combination of skills and personal attributes to the task of leading.

Some health care executives seem to know almost by instinct how to lead, but most become competent leaders by continually learning—by making mistakes, testing out new techniques, refining those techniques that work, and ruling out those that do not. What makes this process successful, however, is a rather mysterious matter. Excellence itself is an elusive quality. We know it when we see it, but trying to pin it down to particular characteristics rarely turns up satisfying answers.

1

What we do know, however, is that health care provides a unique environment and a unique set of challenges for leaders. Many leaders in health care have chosen a career in health services because they believe that their involvement will make a difference. Health care is perceived as being of great value to society, and although increased compensation levels in recent years have made the profession more appealing, many executives are still drawn to health care primarily because they believe in the rewards associated with "service above self." Even those who are not initially "called" to the health care field develop over time an appreciation for the special mission of health services.

The strength of their commitment, however, does not reduce the number of challenges that executives face in the rapidly changing health care environment. Even with all the recent attempts at integration of services, the industry as a whole still functions to a large degree without coordination. It is easy to become consumed with the issues that affect our particular work environment, especially since many institutions and many individuals in health care work in isolation.

Another factor that complicates leadership in health services organizations is the continuing and rapid increase in developments in the technology and science of medicine, which are forcing further divisions and specialization between both physicians and other medical personnel. High-tech specialization, combined with the increasing problem of technical and specialist labor shortages, works against the building of strong team relationships. The contemporary leader in health care must constantly address questions regarding the coordination of services and personnel: Can the internal computer software specialist communicate adequately with the front-line nursing supervisor? Does the "outside" hospital board member understand the dynamics of delivering care in an era when the resource base is eroding?

One of the most significant differences between the health services industry and many other industries is the magnitude of the impact of outcome on patients, medical staff, health services employees, and the community at large. When a patient has been injured by an accident or carelessness in the health setting, the impact is far more severe than when a "five star" restaurant fails to live up to customer expectations. The concern over outcome drives health care providers to work fervently to avoid failure. This is not to suggest that other industries are not driven similarily when the stakes are high, but the results of error in other industries are rarely as visible as they are in health care. In addition, the health care consumer obviously and legitimately anticipates universally high standards in the provision of health care.

Although health services executives may be removed from direct patient care, they are ultimately responsible for the effective delivery of care, as well as the smooth operation of the organization. Neither those who provide care nor those who receive care can tolerate system failure, and it is left to the health care leader to make the system accommodate these high expectations. An organized and effective environment is absolutely essential to outcome and service, yet it is nearly impossible to maintain while juggling such complex demands and circumstances.

Management: Past and Present

Professional management surfaced in the United States in the early 1900s, when structures were simpler and "the boss" was readily identified. As society expanded, the ever-increasing enhancement of technology required more organizational structures. Subsequent succeeding generations of executives witnessed these eras:

1. *Initial organization and structure: 1910 to 1935.* This was an era of growth of new industries and entrepreneurship. It was an era of preregulation and high risk. The health industry was in its organizational infancy. Physicians were individual entrepreneurs. Group practices were limited to a few Mayo-type structures, which were considered controversial and alien in form. Hospitals were individual units, freestanding and independent.

2. *Productivity era: 1935 to 1955.* A science of management began to develop. Units were counted and factories mechanized. World War II had a profound impact on the organization of medicine and how it was delivered. The concept of integrated hospital care matured, and physician practitioners began to focus on activities closer to the hospital.

3. *Systems movement and management control: 1955 to 1970.* Technology continued to advance, and society responded with an endless appetite and a new expectation that medicine and the health system could deliver quality care in limitless quantities. Within hospitals, management engineers were employed to further operational effectiveness. The new organizational charts stressed accountability and the differences between line and staff functions, and planning processes became formalized and structured.

4. *System networking: 1970 to 1980.* Hospitals, group practices, and other providers began to network and link. These linkages, developed initially for sharing resources and services, took on more importance as financial restraints and the regulation of the health industry began to limit decision-making flexibility. There were advantages in joining forces in order to achieve economies of scale

and mutual protection. For-profit hospital systems began to flourish, existing nonprofit systems adopted corporate structure formats and outlook, and independent institutions formed new alliances and consortia.

5. *The new competition: 1980 to 1990.* This was the era of the shakeout and survival of the fittest. High technology, high expectations, and high costs were the drivers for change. Competition was testing the traditional organizational climate. Health organizations responded predictably, similar to other industries that had experienced deregulation and competition. Hospital leaders learned how to "downsize" operations, how to diversify to protect revenue bases, and how to build management teams capable of rapid decision making. In response to these external and internal pressures, organizations created tighter internal control mechanisms and began to seek ways to reward risk takers and innovators. This internal conflict in management direction—over whether to increase bureaucratic control or liberate the decision-making processes—put pressure on the traditional management team and tested the organization's ability to implement crucial change processes.

6. *The present: 1990 to 2000.* Management styles reflect and will continue to reflect a response to economic competition. Management theorists will develop new approaches to help leaders cope in an era that emphasizes the politics of subtraction. Organizations will look for ways to further trim management structures. Top-down bureaucratic control systems will be replaced by highly focused management teams. The art of blending management specialties into highly integrated and interdependent teams will become even more essential.

An age of executive excellence will result from this organizational integration and renewal. Tomorrow's executives will spend more time identifying and rewarding individuals who are risk takers, cultivating innovation and vision rather than merely institutional caretaking.

Lessons from Leaders in Industry

Of course, not everything about health care is unique. We have learned much from business and industry to help us cope with management issues, and we will continue to take our cues from the experiences and successes of our counterparts. For example, the proliferation of bureaucracy in the banking industry in the 1950s and 1960s taught us that organizational bloating combined with a lack of board and management control results in system failures, forced mergers, and restructuring. Like the banking industry, the health industry is awash in stories of restructuring in which corporate headquarters have been downsized to streamline the bureaucracy. The contemporary bank officer is now much more attuned to the needs of the customer. And so are leaders in health care.

Similarly, we have learned from the hotel industry (particularly national chains like Marriott, Hyatt, and Westin) that standardization leads to more consistent and higher-quality services. Of course, most health care organizations must build their reputation for consistent quality regionally or locally, rather than nationally or internationally like the hotel business. Unlike the national hotel chains, we do not have the advantage of being able to instill widespread confidence in quality on the basis of name recognition. But we do understand the importance of quality to consumers (patients), each of whom comes with an individual set of needs, and we know that generating confidence in our ability to serve them creates a loyal patient population.

We have learned other lessons as well—for example, that innovations in management and employee relations in Japanese automobile companies have resulted in greater productivity both in Japan and in the United States, and that with a deliberate compromise on elective procedures, the Canadian health system has succeeded in providing basic health services to all citizens. And we must continue to learn. The most fundamental lesson in all of this is that management excellence is transferable, and if we keep our eye on industry while monitoring the specific needs and changes in the health system, we will develop the tools that we need as we approach the twenty-first century.

But so far we have only addressed the place of leadership in the health care environment. What are the personal and professional attributes that contribute to successful leadership? Most successful leaders seem simply to work very hard at what they do best, bringing themselves and others to new levels of activity and achievement. So how is it that leaders rise from the ranks in the health field? If there is no formula, how can we measure our success? What should we strive for?

Lessons from Leaders in Health Care

It is perhaps most useful, given the assumption that we in health care are at least somewhat unique, to take our cues from some of our own colleagues. Has it been chance when leaders have succeeded in the past? Is there any common thread that links the successes of health care giants like Malcolm MacEachern, George Bugbee, Harry Harwick, Ray Brown, and Stan Nelson? What is it that characterizes their extraordinary contributions?

Malcolm MacEachern was instrumental in the founding of Northwestern University's program in health administration, and he also produced the first definitive textbook on hospital management. MacEachern combined an absolute drive for excellence with an unflagging supply of energy, and he was able to convey his sense of professionalism to those he mentored and sponsored. The MacEachern Board Room at the headquarters of the American College of Healthcare Executives serves as a constant memorial to this outstanding leader and his accomplishments.

George Bugbee may be considered the futurist of the group—quiet, thoughtful, and visionary. He was a builder not only of the American Hospital Association (AHA) but also of the linkages between hospitals and the academic world. His vision contributed to the development of the Association of University Programs in Health Administration (AUPHA), an organization that contributes much to the improvement of curricula in graduate and undergraduate health administration programs. A longtime faculty member at the University of Chicago, and an active writer and researcher, Bugbee developed a lifelong personal network of colleagues and students.

Harry Harwick, the first business manager–executive of the Mayo Clinic, along with the Mayo brothers, successfully nurtured the creation of a group practice where physicians joined together and shared their expertise in an organized structure. The concept of group practice, so common today, was revolutionary in the early 1900s. Harwick's skilled leadership and understanding of the business side of medicine brought physicians, administrators, and other professionals together in a common cause. The American College of Medical Group Administrators (ACMGA) annually awards the Harry J. Harwick Award of Excellence to an administrator selected for "outstanding contributions to the field of health care delivery administration and education." The concepts and values developed by Harwick and his physician colleagues are replicated throughout the nation in major group practices.

Ray Brown, who served as a hospital administrator and professor at the University of Chicago, Duke University, Harvard University, and Northwestern University, is well regarded for his vast understanding of complex operational and human issues. He was a prolific writer and lecturer who could make even the most difficult concepts understandable to the practicing administrator. When Ray was in the room, he was always surrounded by administrators and students who would seek him out for on-the-spot advice and counsel. His clearsightedness and excellent ideas were also valued by professional and political organizations. In addition to serving on a number of national policymaking committees, he served both as president of the American Hospital Association and as a board member of the American College of Hospital Administrators (since 1985, the American College of Healthcare Executives).

Stan Nelson, former chief executive officer of Henry Ford Medical Center in Detroit, Michigan, and former board chairman of the American Hospital Association, will be remembered for his uncanny ability to ask the right question at the right time. He has been able to cut through the issues, focus on the target, and rally colleagues and others to his cause. A builder and supporter of organizations and individuals, he possesses a keen sense of how to deal with governance issues, how to build teams, and how to bring out the best in fellow board members. One of his great tools as a leader is his creative sense of humor.

Were these giants all cut of the same cloth? Indeed not. Although they may have possessed similar virtues—unflagging energy, high ethical standards, and well-defined values—they certainly possessed different personalities. Perhaps the common thread is nothing more than the fact that these leaders found a way, perhaps not even consciously, to fuse personal goals and professional aspirations and responsibilities, and to apply their skills and abilities where they were most needed at the time. Whether deliberately or not, by doing what they did best, they were able to rise to the occasion.

What health care leaders have before them now is certainly a challenge to rise to the occasion. The development of intensive competition in the health industry suggests that new strategies are needed. We have all talked about the hard times, and we have all found various ways to adapt. But even those of us who have weathered the past decade can expect more storms ahead. If the most we can do to prepare is to reexamine the way we lead, the qualities we bring to leadership, and the characteristics that will carry us through the last decade of the century, then that is our ultimate responsibility.

The Leadership Challenge

By the time they reach the executive level, most managers feel quite secure in the knowledge and experience that they have gathered throughout their careers. But now is the time to take another long look at the challenges ahead and to approach the growing demands of the profession with the best tools we can find. For some of us, this will require an attempt to bring traditional leadership skills into balance with the new skills that we need to face contemporary situations. For all of us, it will require an examination of how well we have developed four particular characteristics: balance, direction, flexibility, vision.

These four characteristics or qualities form the basis for the organization of this book; each one is the focus of one of the book's four parts. Within each part, the individual chapters elucidate both the importance of achieving the particular leadership quality, and the issues and challenges involved. (In addition, each chapter begins with a "case in point," an example of how the issues described in the chapter have surfaced in actual practice. Some of the cases are fictitious; others are based on real-life situations.)

The contemporary leader in health care must strive for balance in the use of personal and professional authority and power, knowing when it is appropriate to rely on insight and intuition and when to call on organizational systems to support decisions and activities. Part I, "Balance: The Essence of Health Care Leadership," addresses issues in which balance is an essential element: decision making, ethics, and personal and professional integrity. Whether the leader relies on the power of his or her position in the organization or on the strength derived from personal characteristics and credibility, it is important to use that power with sensitivity. The strong and capable leader knows both how to make authoritative decisions and when to step back and allow others to show their strengths and skills. The ability to weigh personal and professional interests against the increasing needs of staff, patients, the community, and the organization will be one of the measures of excellence in health care leadership in the years to come.

Leaders are also motivated and validated through the respect of their colleagues. They work diligently to earn this respect and not to abuse it—a particularly difficult task in health care, where staff needs and expectations are so widely varied. They also recognize instinctively that lasting results are produced through the work of others and that the foundation of success is teamwork. In directing their staff members, they encourage mutual respect by building productive teams and reinforcing personal and collective achievements. In addition, they work hard to address individual concerns and try to build positive staff relations at all levels of the organization. Part II, "Direction: Leading the Team," focuses on vital issues pertaining to team building and leading in the current health care environment.

Leaders recognize that the goals of the organization will be achieved through the investment of time and energy. They must demonstrate incredible patience and flexibility in working toward those goals, accepting short-term setbacks to ensure that long-range objectives are met. Today's health care leaders must adapt to new organizational systems, economic pressures, and changing staff patterns, taking the responsibility for creating the right conditions for change. Part III, "Flexibility: Adapting to Turbulent Times," addresses the leader's role in adapting to the impending changes in the health care system.

Most leaders are also strongly driven to make a lasting contribution to their organization and their profession. Much energy is expended in trying to leave the organization better off than when they found it. The leader who believes in destiny believes that he or she can make a difference and tries to make decisions that will make the most out of every situation. The chances are that he or she works with a vision in mind, a vision of what the organization would look like if things always went according to plan. Those of us who have devoted most of our careers to attempting to improve a small segment of the health care arena may have a hard time knowing when our work has been completed, or when the challenges have ceased to be exciting and are simply taking their toll on our physical and mental health. Part IV, "Vision: Looking Back and Thinking Ahead," addresses the difficult task of assessing our career from an overall perspective. It is important to be thinking now about the next ten years: When will we have had enough? What do health care organizations and the system as a whole need most from us now? How can we contribute most effectively in the remaining years we plan to spend in the organization? What would we most like to leave behind?

All leaders dislike errors, but most of us are still perpetual optimists. Rather than dwelling on personal or organizational failures, we tend to consider setbacks as "learning experiences." This allows us to develop leadership styles based on what seems to work for us as individuals. When the environment changes, however, as it surely will continue to do, executives have to apply new skills to new situations. To constantly retune and refine management practices to meet current needs is today's health care leadership challenge. Executives who have learned to cultivate self-awareness about their capacity to cope with change and crisis will be the ones who continue to accomplish goals in the face of turbulent times. Those who approach the future with the ability to be balanced, directed, flexible, and visionary will be able to build the bridge to the twenty-first century.

PART I

BALANCE: THE ESSENCE OF HEALTH CARE LEADERSHIP

1

THE DELICATE ART OF DECISION MAKING

Case in Point

John Jackson is the CEO of Midwest Medical Center, a 400-bed hospital with a 70-year history in an urban community. Positioned next door is a large multispeciality clinic of some 225 physicians who admit their patients to several hospitals in the community. The majority of their admissions are to Midwest.

Dr. Rebecca Jones, the president of the group practice, has arranged a confidential meeting with John Jackson. She is concerned that because competition in the community is fierce, physician income is too unstable. She asks whether the hospital would consider a merger with the group practice, explaining that a merger would offer a good opportunity to improve the hospital's market share and to produce efficiencies for both organizations.

John agrees that this is a great idea and tells Dr. Jones that the hospital would be very interested in discussing a merger. Dr. Jones accepts this as a commitment to proceed. Twenty-four hours later, because Dr. Jones has dispatched a memorandum to all of the group physicians, the news of the merger hits the street and John's telephone starts ringing off the hook. A board member calls to suggest that something as important as a merger should have been discussed first by the board. Several physicians who have been regular admitters to the hospital but who are not part of the group practice call to express their anger at the prospect of a merger. They state emphatically that if the merger talks proceed they will move all their patients to the nearest neighboring hospital. John's chief operating officer drops by to report that the hospital is buzzing about the news and asks how the management team should respond to questions.

John Jackson has accidentally created a fire storm. His instincts about the advantages of merging were probably correct, but he lost the game before it even began because he was careless in underestimating the impact the news would have on an unprepared audience. Now that the news is out, he realizes not only that he should have assessed the situation but also that he should have planned the orchestration of his decision-making process. In this case, John will lose credibility in the eyes of his board, members of the medical staff, and his management team. As a seasoned executive, he should have known that the bigger the decision and the more people it affects, the greater the need to prepare the organization for acceptance of the plan.

Much of leadership is an art—the art of knowing when to conform to the norm and when to exert personal influence in the attempt to achieve higher goals. Leaders who understand the importance of this art try to cultivate the intuitive side of managing, learning to trust their instincts as well as the intellectual skills involved in making decisions. They know that the best decisions result from a combination of information and good judgment, and they constantly seek a balance between the two.

Intuition and Information: Finding the Right Mix

Health care executives are expected to make sound decisions based on facts and figures as well as past experiences. Staff members depend on them to provide organizational stability through predictable and consistent decision-making processes. Precisely for this reason, most health care executives are most secure in carrying out decisions when they have taken the time to consider all sides of an issue. But this cautious weighing, while it contributes to stability and measured progress toward a goal, can also lead to excessive bureaucracy. It is particularly difficult for our clinical colleagues, who are often required to marshall facts and make decisions at a moment's notice.

In a field now characterized by volatility and rapid change, health care executives need to make decisions quickly. The stakes are higher and the time line for decision making is usually shorter, so the ability to assess situations quickly and accurately and to draw on decision-making strategies is more dire than ever before. Sometimes in spite of all the reports and position papers that seem to lead to a particular conclusion, the timing for the suggested solution is all wrong. At other times, the external environment may be shifting so rapidly that the whole case has to be reviewed one more time before the solution can be implemented. In other situations, leaders may have to make decisions to act without having completed the customary assessment processes. The optimal conditions for decision making occur when facts are available, issues are weighed, and—with the appropriate use of intuition—the best solution is evident. But needless to say, a lot of decisions get made under less than optimal circumstances.

Executives who work in large hospitals or health systems usually have the advantage of a check-and-balance system, as well as the cooperation of other leaders in the organization, to back up their decisions. There are opportunities to examine processes from different directions, and the wise leader makes use of these opportunities before calling the shots. In smaller organizations, however, where the absence of collegial interchange means that the executive receives little external input, decision making can be a very lonely affair.

But leaders in all organizations face the same dilemma. Knowing when to intervene and make a decision based on instinct, instead of letting the process flow through the organization's decision-making structure, is an ongoing issue for people in positions of authority. How to respond successfully to this issue is one of the mysteries of good leadership. Decisions that are made well—that is, by employing the right combination of intuition and information—can lead to great innovations, in health care as well as in any other field.

Take the case of an urban administrator who discovered that referrals to his downtown center for radiation therapy were declining and then intuitively picked the right time to initiate talks with a suburban competitor. A joint venture was developed by offering radiation therapy at the community hospital and then staffing the program with physicians and technicians from the urban center. In addition to creating expenses and revenue, the venture stabilized market share and strengthened interhospital linkages. The administrator could just as easily have delayed the decision and allowed the community hospital to develop a separate unit, which would only have contributed to the erosion of referrals downtown. But the administrator had the right information and the right instinct to take advantage of the opportunity to act.

Credibility and Innovation in Decision Making

If irrefutable facts suggest a particular outcome, but the leader makes a decision that seems contrary to logic, the leader's judgment is obviously subject to scrutiny. Others in the organization will determine whether or not to support the decision based on their perception of the leader's track record. Leaders therefore must constantly work to enhance their credibility by summoning all possible intellectual, organizational, and creative skills to the task. If an alternate path is chosen, leaders should explain the intent behind the choice so staff members will know that there are good reasons for countering the anticipated process. Wise leaders protect their credibility by being straightforward even when making controversial decisions. Although it is risky to overrule logic in favor of instinct, occasionally such decisions bring about the best results. The trick is to identify those occasions.

The leader's credibility is also enhanced through a continual process of fine-tuning style to meet current organizational needs. Modifying one's style to address a particular problem might short-circuit customary decision-making processes, but this does not necessarily convey a bad message to the organization. As long as the executive guards against exploiting the power of his or her position, a thoughtful change in style might even help to point out ineffective organizational processes, thus contributing to the potential for future innovations.

Imagine a hospital CEO whose associate for professional services is unable to correct or even confront a behavior problem in one of the hospital managers, who has been abrupt and rude to employees. The CEO usually practices a hands-off management style, preferring to delegate authority rather than getting involved in issues that should be handled by members of the management team. However, after all normal approaches (counseling and suggesting approaches to the problem) are exhausted without success, the leader elects to bypass the associate altogether and to confront the manager directly. Before doing so, the CEO discusses the situation with the associate to make sure they agree on the importance of the intended action. The two collaborate and make a joint decision that it is in the best interests of the organization for the leader to intervene.

The process of bypassing the hierarchical structure in the organization creates some interesting dynamics in an already complex interpersonal relationship. But the potential benefit of taking direct action is well worth the risk if the intended outcome (in this case, changing the manager's behavior) is achieved. The CEO is in a position to use the authority of the leadership role to influence the manager's behavior. However, the leader must also avoid any misapplication or misuse of power when addressing the problem. The key to doing this successfully is to maintain credibility and to instill confidence by communicating with both staff members and by clearly defining the roles that both should take. Failure to set up the confrontation on a collaborative basis would have raised the risk that the leader's intervention, while solving the immediate problem, would undermine the trust between the two senior executives.

Being able to deviate from normal procedures to achieve specific objectives is an occasional but very important part of the leader's role. Because the executive in the case above recognized the importance of intervening straightforwardly and deliberately in what normally would have been a matter between two subordinates, it was possible to effectively resolve the ongoing issue. Not intervening might have contributed indirectly to diminished team performance. The leader's awareness that it was time to look beyond the normal channels and to step in to resolve the problem exemplifies the intuitive, even mysterious, aspect of leadership that is so unique to each individual and so difficult to describe.

The Pros and Cons of Organizational Bureaucracy

Most health care executives accept bureaucracy as necessary and inevitable. After all, an effective bureaucracy grapples with ambiguity and uncertainty through established control systems and therefore operates with a wider base of power than is generally granted to most individuals. There is security in knowing that the bureaucracy will counter divided responsibility and attack paternalism through group decision making. So we think of bureaucracy as basically good if it is driven by benevolent motives. By creating interdependent rather than subservient relationships, benevolent bureaucracies acknowledge and promote the idea that the future depends on the performance of all parts and all members of the system.

Bureaucratic systems also work to measure and improve quality.[1] Organizational systems that are driven by the development of data comparing historical performance with current events are inevitably concerned with issues of quality and performance improvement. The movement toward continuous quality improvement that is sweeping the health care field is just one example of the way bureaucratic practices can provide systematic approaches to problem solving.

But it is tyranny—the excess of bureauracy—that should concern us. Tyranny reduces work commitment and destroys individual and professional value systems by taking power out of individuals' hands and depriving them of motivation. The unexpected termination of a staff member by a health services CEO might serve to demonstrate executive power, but it also conveys values that will ultimately destroy team building and effectiveness. Another pervasive and less visible form of tyranny occurs when the executive withholds needed information as a means of testing the employee's ability to arrive at a proper management decision (for example, when the CEO knows that an affected third party has useful data but does not share that knowledge with his or her colleagues).

Excessive bureaucracy threatens organizational ethics and values. It is natural for organizational values to differ, but organizations that focus exclusively on the bottom line, without regard to any other goals, may end up in a state of ethical conflict. In nonprofit health services organizations, where making a profit is not the goal, any "profit" serves only as a means to the end goal of achieving the mission. Similarly, executives of successful for-profit organizations are quite aware that too much focus on the bottom line (and the use of organizational tyranny to improve it) will ultimately be destructive. If the organization has only one goal (that is, turning a profit), the CEO can justify virtually any decision that earns money for the organization. There are no other ethical underpinnings on which to base individual or organizational behavior.

Overdeveloped bureaucracies shield individual managers from personal accountability since responsibility for tough decisions is shared. Although sharing responsibility is an essential part of managing, without a system of personal accountability, responsibility can too easily get shifted around without resolution when things go wrong. For example, an operating room supervisor with no sense of personal accountability could easily avoid a conflict between surgeons and anesthesiologists by dismissing the conflict as an interprofessional problem rather than recognizing it as a scheduling conflict created by the operating room system itself. More than once in the world of business bureaucracy, capable and trusting managers have been maneuvered into serving as scapegoats for one another's decisions. In these situations, a manager may "behave like Attila the Hun, but if [the manager] contributes substantially to organizational effectiveness, all is forgiven."[2]

Organizational bureaucracy tends to breed conformity, which contributes to corporate culture but may inhibit individual growth. If asked to comment on how things really work in a large health care system, middle managers (such as chief radiology technologists, supervisors of the medical records department, or operating room or nursing unit managers) would often give responses like the following:

- "Key issues always seem to require group input. Why doesn't someone simply make a decision?"
- "There are days when I think that the reward system depends more on my social accountability than on what I really accomplish. My social behavior in group meetings is important. My superior's jokes are more important than my own."
- "If I really want to confront someone because I believe they're wrong, the team doesn't like it. Everyone around here avoids head-on confrontation. We go around smiling even when we're hurting."

By fostering widespread conformity and dependence, zealous bureaucrats can easily reinforce their own power base, taking advantage of the willingness of staff members to work as a team. They know that an atmosphere of conformity discourages individuals from rocking the boat or acting on their own ideas.

All CEOs must unbundle and delegate responsibilities so their time can be spent on strategic issues. But CEOs who practice tyrannical bureaucracy have other motives for delegation and unbundling: to keep their options open, minimize personal risk, and distance themselves from error. Unscrupulous CEOs might even send inadequate instructions to their staff and then back away to watch what happens. They are willing to send the whole organization off in the wrong direction so they can step in at the last minute and play the hero by saving the organization from disaster.

Such situations are extreme, but the point is that when bureaucracy is out of control, unsupported by an ethical basis for operation, there is inherent potential for misuse of the leadership role. The leader's responsibility is to employ the best that organizational bureaucracy has to offer—a structure for making and supporting important decisions—without using it to stifle individuals' innovations or avoid personal accountability. Leaders who want to encourage innovation and creative decision making, in themselves and their staff, will build teams that can function effectively in the organizational structure without compromising individual autonomy. (The team-building process is addressed in Part II.)

Principles of Decision Making in Bureaucratic Organizations

Working within the organizational bureaucracy, leaders should base their decision-making strategies on three basic principles. First, leaders must believe in process, even though they know that the usual procedures do not work to resolve every critical situation. Decision-making processes must be functional, derived to address daily issues and occurrences. The leader who believes in process will also be better equipped for situations that call for unconventional approaches.

The second principle is to look for the "wild card" when making decisions on key issues. The wild card is the instinct for the right time to act (or not to act) in spite of data that indicate the contrary. The ability to recognize and trust this instinct is one of the unique characteristics of real leaders. Willingness to consider and act on unconventional approaches often stimulates organizational innovation. Leaders who believe in the action they are taking are able to rally the organization by encouraging them to stretch a little further. As a result, management staff and others are able to see that they possess more potential than they had imagined. For example, a leader who has had to reduce expenses and downsize the organization, but who then finds an opportunity to take on a needed community service, sends the message that the organization has begun to heal.

The third principle is that the usual and customary approaches to decision making sometimes have to be challenged and set aside, even if straying from the norm seems like a risky proposition. The opportunity to set aside convention will test the strength and flexibility of management teams. It might ruffle a few feathers in the process, but it will usually lead to improved decision making in the future, as well as to the successful outcome of the situation at hand.

Organizations stagnate in the absence of creative decision making. Although the organizational structure should always be designed to support efficient and effective decision-making processes, it should also allow the leader to take full responsibility for determining how to make the best decision in the most timely fashion. Developing an environment of trust within a team and providing team members room to grow is part of that responsibility. Good teams usually make good decisions. The leader who believes in the team's ability will enable the group to make decisions without encouraging "group think," a process in which team members agree with the leader in spite of their better sense. Confident leaders who have faith in the contributions the team can make will create an open atmosphere that permits discussion and debate.

Leadership Goals for Artful Decision Makers

Finding the right balance between conventional and unconventional approaches to decision making, between individual and bureaucratic control, and between withholding and exerting personal authority is a never-ending process. Most of us have tried numerous decision-making strategies with varying degrees of success. Although different approaches work for different people, the most successful decision makers work with several principles in mind.

First, building teams is the best way to discourage turf guarding and to ensure that decisions are accepted throughout the organization. Organizations that pride themselves on team building eliminate any reason for divisional managers to build protective walls around their responsibilities or to discourage communication between teams. Allowing divisional directors to drive the decision-making process can be unhealthy, even destructive, if it leads to an overly competitive environment. The very nature of team building is such that it recognizes group more than individual effort. Thus, in a mature and fully functional team, peer pressure should make it difficult for a single individual to impede the group's progress by holding back vital information or otherwise operating in a dysfunctional fashion.

Second, allowing staff members to make mistakes is the best way for them to learn and build confidence in their own decision-making abilities. If you do not allow a certain amount of error, employees will become overly cautious, unable to take even well-considered risks for fear of committing the slightest error. Executives need to make it clear that they are willing to take the heat for mistakes made by less-experienced staff. They should see to it that staff members are never in a position of being unprotected in organizational confrontations.

Backing up staff decision making does not give the leader license to demand a reciprocal relationship. CEOs who encourage their staff to be loyal to them rather than the organization (by taking the attitude that "I'll protect you, but you had better protect me") are undermining the foundation of the relationship. In addition, CEOs who tell employees that mistakes are okay but then use the mistakes to justify dismissals or transfers are guilty of entrapment. Professional executives must be sensitive when applying the tools of their trade so as to ensure a benevolent, well-managed bureaucracy. Being willing to take the heat can be a lonely position.

Third, to create order out of chaos, health care leaders sometimes have to function autocratically. Effective leaders realize this. They know what is best for their organizations, and they are able to assume different roles to meet shifting organizational needs. Ineffective leaders also shift roles, but they are more likely to use a tyrannical style that is arbitrary, capricious, and confusing to employees.

Finally, the way the leader is perceived is very influential in determining the extent to which decisions are accepted and supported by staff. Be conscious of the image you project. In any organization, employees pick up clues about their CEO and about how the CEO perceives them. Well-intentioned executives should be conscious of this vigilance and of how they are perceived by members of the board, the medical staff, fellow executives, employees, and the community. Some CEOs might be surprised at what they discover.

In thinking about the image you project, it might be helpful to honestly consider questions like these: How accessible am I? Do I contribute to the preservation of the organizational culture, or do I try to develop a personal cult? Am I arrogant or friendly in communications with fellow professionals, particularly those I do not know? Do employees fear me or trust me? Have I stood up for the right of the individual who has been intentionally or accidentally wronged by the system? Your answers to such questions reveal a lot about your image and probably about your credibility with staff.

Responsibility: The Buck Stops Here

Since the early 1980s, it has seemed more and more obvious that organizational commitment will not flourish in a workplace dominated by traditional models of control. Managers who want to do well need to rethink their relationships with their workers. Bureaucracies must be monitored to ensure that they are benevolent and that they work to secure moral and ethical values. Controlling a bureaucracy requires an executive who can create and maintain management approaches—including skilled decision making—that are sensitive to the environment but that also maximize the commitment and involvement of employees, managers, boards, and physicians.

In a complex health care system, the ultimate decision making responsibility falls to the leader. Executives must oversee many organizational functions to ensure that patients receive appropriate care. If we stop short of taking full responsibility, things go wrong and people are hurt. A chief executive officer who is unwilling to confront a situation involving an impaired physician jeopardizes both the patient and the organization. Making the right decision for the organization can sometimes mean facing conflicts between our dedication to individuals and our greater responsibility to the organization.

The delicate art of decision making—the ability to rely on solid information, yet draw on the power of intuition—is only effective as long as the organization's goals and interests are kept in mind. It is up to health care leaders to monitor value systems, promote and protect the corporate culture, and avoid the personal pitfalls that go hand in hand with an overdeveloped ego. If we can build an organization that meets its organizational and societal goals, we have faced our responsibility head on—with character, intelligence, and a benevolent spirit.

Notes

1. A. Ross, "Healthcare Executives: Are We Benevolent Bureaucrats?" *Healthcare Executive* 1, no. 6 (1986): 40–43.
2. W. G. Scott and D. K. Hart, *Organizational America* (Boston: Houghton Mifflin, 1979).

2

ETHICS AND THE CEO: MAKING MISSION MATTER

It hadn't been a good year financially for Mid-Central Memorial. The bottom line was eroding and the net profit of this 500-bed hospital was 2 percent, down from the previous year's 3.4 percent. Although management staff had been working diligently to reduce expenses, fluctuations in volume were still causing a problem. Management of DRGs was working well, thanks to a cooperative medical staff, but neighboring hospitals were cutting back in response to weakening patient volume. Charity care write-offs were increasing, although still at a manageable rate.

The hospital's CEO, Helen Weisman, was very concerned. At the most recent meeting of the board of directors, the chairman of the finance committee had suggested that it was time to eliminate a few of the hospital's low-margin programs. One of the programs that might be affected by programmatic cutbacks was the one supporting a newly opened 45-bed off-campus AIDS hospice unit, which Mid-Central Memorial operated as a community service. The unit had received widespread community support but there were concerns that the sponsorship of the project might attract additional AIDS patients to the hospital, which would bring further financial strain.

The hospice unit was being subsidized by Mid-Central Memorial by only $120,000 per year, but because of the perceived risks to the staff of providing care for additional AIDS patients, opponents of the unit were focusing on its financial viability as a means of urging Mid-Central out of this "loss leader."

Fortunately for both the hospital and the community, the board, medical staff, and management had recently gone through an extensive update of the hospital's strategic plan, including a major rewriting (and adoption) of a mission statement stressing the hospital's commitment to meeting the needs of the underserved. AIDS patients obviously were part of this segment of the population.

Helen Weisman was able to use this updated and well-endorsed mission statement as a means of reminding board members, and critics among the medical staff and management, that continuing the support of the AIDS hospice was essential to the hospital's mission—a position that was strongly supported by the entire hospital board and most of its medical staff. Helen knew that in the absence of this mission statement, the program might not have survived. Keeping the focus on the mission made the difference.

Although most health care leaders are familiar with the bioethical issues that have dominated the health care arena in recent years, many of us lag behind in our understanding of ethical issues related to business practices. In the absence of formal training in ethics, we tend to "wing it," relying on instinct and drawing on previous experience to point us in the right direction. Although most of our instincts are probably on target most of the time, generally we are poorly prepared to answer complex ethical questions. This chapter addresses some of the challenges health care leaders must face in establishing a strong ethical basis for operation in the health care organization.

We have not always had very good examples to follow. Individual and corporate ethical misconduct has been highly publicized, leading some to suggest that such behavior—that is, compromising organizational integrity for personal gain, sometimes even in violation of the law—is an inevitable, seemingly contagious by-product of competition. Even more alarming is the way that so-called leaders in the business community have been able to rationalize their unethical behavior, believing wholeheartedly that the activity they were engaged in was not really illegal or immoral. Recent wrongdoing among government officials seems to reinforce the idea that no organization is exempt from these problems.

Perhaps we should feel good about the fact that in a recent survey, 63 percent of the business leaders interviewed said that a company is stronger if it maintains high ethical standards.[1] But the implication of the flip side of this statistic is that 37 percent of the business leaders do *not* believe that maintaining high ethical standards necessarily adds to a company's strength. If that many leaders consider adherence to ethical standards as inconsequential in determining a company's ability to succeed, perhaps it is not so surprising that so many are willing to compete without regard to ethical behavior.

Competition and Ethics in Health Care

The health services industry has been propelled into a highly competitive environment without much time to prepare itself to contend with every-day business ethics and values. Unbridled competition in the absence of established rules of conduct can foster some very peculiar behavior. We are fortunate that we and our colleagues in the health care field probably come to our professions with a fairly well developed sense of proper ethical be-havior. Most of us have chosen to become involved in patient care because we are at least somewhat service minded. When we do have to wing it, we draw on the same set of personal ethical standards and values that drove us into health care in the first place. We draw on the lessons learned from early personal experiences with ethical decision making, as well as from experi-ences in academic or religious settings, to lead us to the "right" decisions and actions.

But to keep pace with the influence of competition on health care, health care leaders must take a more decisive step toward etablishing organization-wide standards and expectations regarding values and ethics. Responsive leadership is the key to ensuring ethical behavior in any orga-nization. Health care executives have the difficult task of making sure that their organization not only espouses ethical standards but instills them in the corporate culture so they will be passed on to individuals. Obviously, this is a difficult thing to do, but the leader who accepts the burden of this respon-sibility will benefit from the challenge of contributing to and preserving the integrity of the organization.

Leadership Ethics and Standards

Health care leaders must lead by example, and to do so they must set their own standards for proper conduct. They must know how far they are will-ing to stretch rules, for themselves and for others; what to do if and when organizational goals compromise their personal standards, and vice versa; and when to confront unethical personal and professional behavior in staff members. As part of this responsibility, executives must be careful to avoid preferential treatment of staff. In appreciation of services well performed, some executives reward immediate subordinates very liberally, without realizing that other staff who are performing equally well in other parts of the organization might feel slighted. CEOs who are willing to undermine the equitable compensation of individuals throughout the organization have not fully accepted their overriding responsibility to act fairly. Compromising this responsibility might reflect an urge to purchase personal loyalty by granting special privileges—a dangerous characteristic in anyone who expects to be a credible leader.

If they have not examined their own expectations and standards on a personal level, health care executives will not be prepared for challenges with staff members. As the guardians of ethical conduct, health care leaders face daily decisions about whether or not to address individuals' behavior and what measures to take if they do. Consider, for example, the following scenarios:

1. Suppose a prominent member of your medical staff sends an insulting memo to one of your hospital managers. This physician is responsible for admitting many patients to your hospital each year. What should you do?

2. Suppose an administrative assistant who is responsible for physician recruitment quietly sets himself up in a real estate business. When showing prospective physician candidates around town, he refers them to specific realtors and receives part of the commission on sales in return. Why is this wrong?

3. Suppose a surgeon with a temper throws instruments in the operating room. You hear of it. The chief of surgery is unwilling to confront the situation. What do you do?

4. Suppose a board member who heads a large construction firm takes you aside quietly and tells you that he has worked very hard for years on behalf of the hospital and hopes that this will help you make the correct decision in selecting the contractor for the next hospital job. How do you deal with this?

5. Suppose you find that one of your administrators has pushed through a much larger salary increase for her secretary than the levels established through usual market surveys and that this has created an inequity for others in the same category. How do you resolve this?

6. Suppose you are the chief executive officer in a major teaching hospital. You hear a rumor that there are so many "no codes" that the residents are fretting because they are not getting sufficient experience in resuscitating patients. And then you receive a letter from

a patient's family that indicates that in spite of their clearly documented wish that their father not be resuscitated, the medical staff did resuscitate him and he was left to linger painfully for another 24 hours. Is this an ethical issue or just a matter of circumstance, and what do you do about it?

A leader's inclination to look the other way on little things, even more than on larger organizational issues, contributes to declining staff confidence in ethics and values. A CEO who is unwilling to really confront poor behavior in others is putting both the leadership position and the internal structure of the organization at tremendous risk. In addition, executives who set one ethical standard for the organization and another for themselves deserve to experience what will ultimately follow: the erosion of self-respect and, potentially, the loss of the privilege of leadership. When dealing with human life, these ethical considerations become increasingly complex, and the implications of ethical decision making are far-reaching. It is imperative that health care leaders examine and define for themselves where they stand on ethical issues.

Ethical Frameworks

Most well-intentioned executives approach ethical decisions from one of two theoretical positions. Those who ascribe to a utilitarian perspective tend to make judgments based on what provides the greatest good for the greatest number of people. The utilitarian leader in the health setting would opt for rigid policies and procedures, considering them to be ethically justifiable because they benefit all of the patients served. In the case of a physician violation of medical staff policy, for example, the hospital board with a utilitarian administrator would elect to give the physician a temporary suspension rather than a mild reprimand, on the premise that the policy was implemented for the good of all members of the medical staff and must be followed totally consistently.

Other leaders tend to emphasize the right of the individual (a Kantian orientation) over good for the greatest number. These leaders would try to stop a train if it looked like an individual would be run over. In the case of the delinquent physician, an administrator who was a strong advocate for individualism might take extra measures to prevent action against the physician. The individual's needs would take precedence over responsibility to the whole organization. The administrator might be inclined to give the physician the benefit of the doubt and a second chance to do things right.

Although there are certainly many other ethical perspectives to add to and complicate decision making, most executives align themselves broadly with one or the other of these two perspectives. Differences in leadership styles are based in part on which of the views leaders adopt and how consciously they adhere to it. Understanding the nature of the two different orientations may help you to explain why your colleagues process the same information that you do and yet arrive at a different solution to the problem.

Mission: Preserving Ethics and Standards in the Organization

The ethical challenges are greater when dealing with the conflicting goals, values, and interests of the staff and organization. When working with teams, leaders must not only hold fast to their own values and beliefs but also balance individual and staff interests. The leader is forced to weigh individual needs and potential against what will work best for the team as a whole. It is important for leaders to cultivate a corporate culture in which organizational values are widely known, and to establish organizational guidelines that can be called upon when ethical issues arise throughout the organization. Although the leaders are the guardians of the organization's ethics, they should not be left alone to defend the actions solely on the basis of their own values and standards. Everyone in the organization should be equipped to exercise good judgment based on the organization's ethics and standards.

The CEO's greatest source of support in preserving ethical conduct within the organization is the organizational mission. A clearly stated mission helps to determine the ethical underpinnings of the organization and to define the legitimate use of power to accomplish organizational goals. Staff members who understand and internalize the organization's mission will have a sense of purpose and direction, which should increase their motivation as well as their ethical decision-making power.

The Mission Statement

To verify its purpose and direction, the organization needs a meaningful mission statement. The mission statement is a vital means of communicating to all members of an enterprise what the organization is all about. When designed and adopted by all the members of the organization's teams, the statement helps to build morale and to guide leaders and staff through difficult decisions. A meaningful statement supports and encourages change by articulating the organization's evolving vision of itself. An example of an organizational mission statement is shown in Exhibit 2.1.

Mission statements should be carefully crafted in understandable terms. The goal is to end up with objectives that can be articulated by employees

Exhibit 2.1 Mission Statement Virginia Mason Medical Center

Virginia Mason will provide the finest health care possible for our patients. This commitment is the basis for all we do.

We believe that professional excellence combined with staff collaboration, integration, and teamwork results in the very best health care.

We strongly support medical education and research to ensure that our patients benefit from the most effective advances in medical care.

We will share in the responsibility of providing health care for the poor, disadvantaged, and medically underserved.

---

at every level in the organization—not necessarily word for word but by concept and purpose. Employee orientation programs provide an excellent opportunity to carefully explain the organization's mission (in fact, programs that provide only a cursory presentation of the mission statement really sell themselves short).

Many mission statements have been developed by one or two executives and then endorsed by a compliant board. Mission statements derived from this process tend to be lifeless because they do not reflect either the organizational culture or the reality of daily work in the organization. When conducted well, the preparation of a mission statement can and should be a synergistic, team-building process; when shortcuts are taken, it is a useless exercise.

Putting Mission into Practice

Let's explore some guidelines for making sure that your organization is properly addressing the issues of ethics, values, and social responsibility. After all, the leader needs an overall sense of roles and responsibilities if the organization's mission is to be of value.

The role of the CEO. It is important to remember, first, that the primary responsibility for upholding ethics falls to the leader. The leader (along with the management team) is responsible for energizing the organization and introducing it to its responsibilities for ethical and social behavior. The role of the CEO in this regard is more important than that of either the board or the medical staff because the CEO and the management team provide on-site visibility. They set the tone for the organization on a day-to-day basis and are therefore able to make lasting changes. Leaders influence outcome by establishing the organizational structure (that is, the benevolent bureacracy) that will make things happen.

Despite the implications of the highly publicized CEO turnover rates, effective leadership is still the health system's best hope for anchoring ethics, values, and social responsibility within organizations. The CEO nurtures the organizational social conscience by being personally dedicated and committed to accomplishing an organizational mission based on good ethical conduct. The CEO creates the example through persistence and consistent personal performance and through a personal understanding of individual and organizational strengths and weaknesses. By setting a personal example, the executive promotes ethical decision making throughout the health care setting.

Team responsibility. Executives should surround themselves with people who are knowledgeable and strong enough to take some personal risks in order to do the job right. In their efforts to build a responsible team, CEOs should foster a toughness of spirit that encourages individuals to stretch and provides the courage to cope, to make a difference, and to discover and build a sense of purpose in their work.

Medical staff members are an essential part of this team. Although physicians may not always agree with or naturally identify with broader organizational issues, they are generally in a perfect position to represent the rights of the patients and the medical staff. They offer a perspective that the executive needs and may not be able to gather in any other way.

The governing board also has a vital role in monitoring ethics, values, and social behavior, but the amount of time that board members can spend in the health care environment is limited. In addition, some trustees encounter difficulties in translating business practices into the health services environment. For example, a business executive trustee who demands bottom-line performance of the hospital executive, even at the risk of undermining the organization's responsibility to care for the underserved, does not have the full range of knowledge of the health care setting that is needed to accurately represent the organization's interests. The CEO depends on the board's input and decision-making skills and counts on board members to support the organization's mission, although they do not carry the primary responsibility for ensuring ethical conduct.

Supporting staff. Maintaining consistent and equitable relations with staff greatly enhances the leader's ability to influence ethics in the organization. Listed below are a few concrete suggestions for reinforcing staff and recognizing their contributions:

1. Pay close attention to internal recognition events, such as retirements, tenure teas, and so on, to let staff know that *you* think their contribution to the organization is important.

2. Work hard to ensure that employees who leave the organization are well placed elsewhere.

3. Walk around to see what staff members are doing, but try not to surprise them.

4. Really maintain an open-door policy for staff who want to consult with you. Always respect confidences.

5. Never overlook regular performance appraisals for your staff. It is easy to forget that something that is a routine practice for you is an important annual event for the team member being reviewed.

6. Seek out reverse appraisals by asking your staff to evaluate you. Your personal reputation should be beyond reproach but should not shelter you from feedback from staff.

7. Use meeting times and management decision-making sessions as opportunities to inject information and encourage dialogue about ethical issues and conduct in the organization.

Statement of values. The leader's goal in encouraging awareness of the mission is to build a team that has the courage of its convictions. The team should be able to identify the principles that drive the organization toward its goals. The health care leader should work with board and staff members to articulate statements about these principles that can be formed into a statement of values. The statement of values complements the mission statement by focusing on internal values. It is most useful in prescribing acceptable organizational behavior—that is, in establishing a code of conduct. The following examples from Kenneth Blanchard and Norman Vincent Peale's *The Power of Ethical Management* illustrate the kinds of statements the leader is looking for in developing a values statement:

- *Purpose.* The mission of our organization is communicated from the top. Our organization is driven by values, hopes, and a vision that helps us to determine what is acceptable and unacceptable behavior.

- *Pride.* We feel proud of ourselves and of our organization. We know that when we feel this way, we can resist temptation to behave unethically.

- *Patience.* We believe that holding to our ethical values will lead us to success in the long term. This involves maintaining a balance between caring about results and caring about how we achieve these results.

- *Persistence.* We have a commitment to live by ethical principles. We are committed to this commitment. We make sure our actions are consistent with our purpose.

- *Perspective.* Our managers and employees take time to pause and reflect, take stock of where we are, evaluate where we are going, and determine how we are going to get there.[2]

Like the mission statement, the statement of values must be more than a superficial document and should be developed with the involvement of participants in the organization. Team members must contribute to the development of the statement if it is going to reflect the team's guiding operating principles. The CEO must be careful not to assume that a well-written values statement has been accepted by the management staff and others until there is open discussion of and consensus reached on the key principles included. The resulting statement should be clear and succinct, representing a unified perspective on the beliefs that characterize the organization (see Exhibit 2.2).

Exhibit 2.2   Sample Values Statement

Our health care is distinguished by our tradition of values that characterize all we are and aspire to be.

Service
We deliver personalized service to our patients. This includes compassion and respect for the patient and a constant striving to achieve the ideal in health care service. In all that we do, the patient comes first.

Excellence
We define excellence as combining skill, innovation, creativity, professionalism and compassion. We expect this excellence of all our staff, believing that it is an essential part of patient care, education and research. As part of our commitment to excellence, we provide health care value. We achieve this through cost-effective medical practice, operating efficiency, and sound financial management.

Teamwork
We adhere to a professional and personal code of conduct in which teamwork is the essential characteristic. We combine excellence and a multidisciplinary approach in providing care for our patients.

Integrity
We demonstrate the highest levels of ethical and professional conduct in a place of healing, caring, teaching, and research. We recognize the worth and dignity of the individual in our relationships with patients and families, our co-workers, and our community.

The Challenge to Health Care Leaders

When resolving ethical questions, you may not always know whether the decision you are making is the right one. There may come a point at which you cannot afford to deliberate any further, and you must make a decision and hope you can live with it. The questions listed below were designed by Laura Nash to assist with ethical decision making. Your responses may help you to clarify your reasons for making the decision you made. If you feel comfortable with your answers, you have probably made the best decision you can make under the circumstances.

1. Have you defined the problem accurately?
2. How would you define the problem if you stood on the other side of the fence?
3. How did this situation occur in the first place?
4. To whom and to what do you give your loyalty as a person and as a member of the corporation?
5. What is your intention in making this decision?
6. How does this intention compare with the probable results?
7. Whom could your decision or action injure?
8. Can you discuss the decision with the affected parties before making the decision?
9. Are you confident that your decision will be as valid over a long period of time as it seems now?
10. Could you discuss without qualm your decision or action to your boss, your CEO, the board of directors, your family, and society as a whole?
11. What is the symbolic potential of your action if understood? If misunderstood?
12. Under what conditions would you allow exceptions to your stand?[3]

Conclusion

Fortunately, more and more resources are becoming available for assistance in working through these tough ethical issues in the health care setting. Professional libraries in organizations such as the American College of Healthcare Executives and the Medical Group Management Association (MGMA) are excellent sources of current articles. Most graduate programs in health administration provide courses on business ethics. In addition, networking with colleagues who encounter similar problems is one of the best means of identifying the issues and sorting out ethical options. There is also a growing cadre of ethics consultants who specialize in health care.

Of course, before seeking help the leader must first recognize that the problem he or she is addressing is one that involves ethical issues. The first and most important source of help then comes from within: the leader must recognize the real issue and identify it as one involving questions of "right" and "wrong." Once the problem has been identified as an ethical issue, help can be sought more readily.

Notes

1. "Business Leader Survey," *Seattle Post-Intelligencer*, February 6, 1990, B2.
2. K. Blanchard and N. V. Peale, *The Power of Ethical Management* (New York: William Morrow, 1988), 125.
3. L. Nash, "Ethics without a Sermon: Ethics and Practice," in *Managing the Moral Corporation* (Boston: Harvard Business Review, 1989), 245.

3

LEADERSHIP INTEGRITY: RECONCILING PERSONAL INTERESTS AND PROFESSIONAL RESPONSIBILITY

Case in Point

Years ago I asked a seasoned and well-respected health care leader to relate one of the tougher decisions he had made during his career. He surprised me by focusing on an incident involving only one staff member.

In his first job after graduate school, my friend inherited the medical records department as one of the departments he was expected to supervise in a group practice organization. Early on he learned that the department was in a mess. Medical records were seldom delivered in time for patient appointments, so the medical staff was in constant turmoil. A quick study of the circumstances revealed that the reason for the chaos was the department manager's lack of managerial expertise and leadership.

But what to do? The manager had been in the position for a long time, and although the organization had increased in size, the manager had not grown in her capacity to manage or lead. To compound the problem, no one had been willing to confront the manager's poor performance, in part because no one wanted to add to her already difficult personal circumstances (she was a widow with six dependent children). Yet the department was a shambles. The manager seldom came to work on time. There was a constant stream of excuses. Good employees were leaving the organization, but no one would confront the problem.

The administrator checked carefully to make sure that the organization had truly tried to resolve the problem through counseling and timely written warnings. At one point the personnel record even revealed that the employee had been placed on probation. Still no one would take the final action that was needed so badly.

My administrator friend decided the manager had to go. He arranged a decent separation package and notified her of her termination. Then he prepared for the onslaught of anger from the medical staff and employees, who he expected would be outraged at the action.

Nothing happened. No one objected. Many breathed a sigh of relief, and most wondered why the action had not been taken earlier. My friend learned that incompetence is often tolerated less well by fellow employees than by the boss. Although he was not comfortable personally with the action he had to take, he knew the action was absolutely necessary for the organization. To this day, however, the executive remembers the importance of working the problem out in a compassionate fashion. No quick, middle-of-the-night termination was involved because he appreciated the importance of a humane approach to a difficult problem.

Health care executives know that no two days are the same. Schedules change constantly, as do the challenges and problems encountered along the way. On one day the leader may be involved in working out a severance package for clinic manager who has to be separated from the organization because of expense reductions, and on the next day the leader may be involved in initiating planning for a major revision of the institution's long-range plan. The leader must be able to respond to the need to be flexible while continuing to monitor and measure day-to-day events.

As the central figure responsible for marshaling human and other resources to fuel the organization, the health care leader must be committed to organizational goals without letting personal feelings or interests get in the way. This becomes a challenge if the demands of the organization push the leader to the point of compromise on personal standards or beliefs. A hospital CEO who knows that a member of the board is pushing a particular program only because it will result in personal financial gain is in a precarious position. The situation will have to be handled sensitively, yet expeditiously, to avoid undermining the leader's personal values and integrity. When confronted with this type of situation, inexperienced leaders may buckle, either unable to meet their responsibility to the organization or unable to maintain a sense of integrity about what they are expected to do. With more experience, however, they begin to define for themselves the ways in which their personal goals mesh with the goals of the organization and, conversely, the ways in which they are unable or unwilling to compromise personal beliefs to fulfill their responsibility to the organization. Establishing and adhering to a personal and professional code of ethics enables the leader to approach such conflicts with a sense of balance, with a solid and well-thought-out foundation for action.

We expect leaders to possess skill, judgment, initiative, and overall technical and social competence. But can we expect that these characteristics alone will give them the singlemindedness to fulfill their responsibilities without sometimes being distracted by their own goals or interests? No matter how many traditional leadership traits they possess, leaders who refuse to look closely and honestly at their own interests and biases will have a difficult time if they find themselves at odds with the organization. Leaders must operate from a fundamental base of honesty—with themselves, and with colleagues and others in the organization.

Sometimes responsibility to the organization does require personal compromise, but it is important to distinguish between compromising our personal preferences and compromising our personal beliefs or goals. We have all found ourselves in situations where we had to do things we did not particularly like or want to do. Perhaps we were called upon to resolve a conflict we would have preferred to avoid, or to confront behavior we would have preferred to ignore. To deal with those situations effectively, we have had to push ourselves, knowing that by confronting an issue directly we were not only fulfilling our obligations to the organization but ultimately contributing to our own effectiveness as leaders as well. If choosing to act is consistent with our personal beliefs, then perhaps what we have to overcome is not so much a compromise of our integrity but a challenge to our leadership style.

The Dynamics of Leadership

Health care leaders often need to balance complex needs and interests—their own, their staff's, and their organization's. They must not only be aware of these dynamics but also have the strength and insight to address any conflicts that arise. Keeping all of these demands in perspective takes a tremendous amount of coordination, which even the most effective leaders have to cultivate consciously throughout their careers. The responsibilities outlined in the rest of this chapter are among those that create the most complex dynamics and challenges for leaders.

Maintaining Distance

The health care leader must view the environment from a distance in order to be objective about the organization's operations. The CEO who becomes too close to the chief operating officer (or any other colleague) might have difficulty when directing, correcting, or motivating that same staff member. Sharing concerns and problems with subordinates, particularly without discretion, can easily lead to a perception within the organization that you are an uncertain leader, so it is important to have the presence of mind to keep the distance needed to make decisions and take appropriate action. Close friendships with staff can make it more difficult for the leader to confront tough choices and make objective decisions, particularly when the outcome of a decision could affect the friendships. Just as the captain of a ship endures a solitary voyage, the leader of a health care organization must be able to tolerate some isolation and even loneliness.

We have probably all had times when we would have preferred to be one of the followers instead of having to take the leadership position. It sometimes appears that turf is better defined and collegial relationships are easier among staff who have less authority. But it is more likely that, because they have less authority to change things, these staff members simply rely on each other for support. Recognizing and accepting the importance of the leadership role means being willing to sacrifice some of that camaraderie because you want to (and can) make decisions that improve the whole organization. As much as we may sometimes feel inclined to be part of the gang, we must guard against compromising the authority of our role as leaders. An effective leader is able to join in and celebrate the efforts of the team but still keep a certain distance from the individual players.

Keeping the Right People in the Right Jobs

Sometimes the responsibility for marshaling resources where they are needed involves making difficult decisions regarding changes in staff positions. When such changes affect the makeup of the the management team, the leader is in a stressful position. Dismissing a marginal performer is a difficult task, but it does not compare to the agony of moving out a competent colleague who simply cannot meet the changing needs of the organization. It can be torturous to try to articulate the reason for the termination, particularly if the colleague has performed competently. If measures taken to retrain the individual have been unsuccessful, the CEO is likely to feel responsible for the failure. For terminated employees, the sense of failure is obviously even worse, particularly if they have done everything that was expected and assigned. Being terminated under such circumstances by someone perceived to be a friend or counselor is extremely painful and may be damaging to an individual's self-confidence.

But the leader is responsible to both the individual and the organization. The end result of the action (the separation) may, in fact, work out better than anticipated for both parties if care has been taken to counsel the employee carefully, to provide a fair separation package, and to honestly explain the reason for the separation. The final task for the leader is to pull out all the stops and help the individual relocate. Too many leaders fall short in this respect.

Keeping a Flexible Leadership Style

Leadership style usually evolves in response to the changing needs of the organization. A style focusing on consensus building, for example, would probably work well in a hospital or group practice that has a history of stability and is humming along with a good bottom line and a content and mature staff. However, the same organization would fare less well under this type of leadership if there were a crisis and decisions suddenly needed to be made with expediency and with some risk to an eroding bottom line. More decisiveness and less democracy might be needed temporarily to resolve the critical issue of the day.

Leadership styles must change in moments of crisis. Although some health care leaders may not be comfortable with the idea of changing styles to meet current demands, preferring instead to rely on tried-and-true methods of leadership, they will continue to be confronted in the next decade with situations in which a new approach will be the only way to direct the organization successfully. Flexibility is an essential component of leading in the changing health care environment. It is not, however, always easy to achieve. The leader's style has usually developed over years of practice at responding to similar situations. But sometimes what seem like similar cases are not alike at all, and taking a different approach to problem solving might work best. Leaders should be conscious of their tendency to revert to past practices and to try instead to be open to varying their approach.

Monitoring Decision Making

When it comes to making decisions, the buck does stop at the top. The leader is responsible for seeing that decisions get made in a timely fashion, but this does not mean that all decisions should be made at the top. In fact, most decisions should be made at lower levels in the organization.

The leader has to be in touch with what is going on in all departments of the hospital or health care organization, and must delegate decision making to the appropriate level. This means keeping channels of communication open with all staff. If news of a financial setback does not reach the executive level of the health care organization because a manager of a department believes that bad news is not welcome, the management team has a serious problem that will require urgent attention. The wise leader keeps in touch to avoid such occurrences and encourages managers to support communication within and between their staff teams. The importance of regular medical staff briefings to support the free exchange of timely information cannot be overemphasized. Through meetings and other monitoring measures, leaders keep an eye on the target without getting lost in detail. They keep their staff motivated by delegating decision-making responsibility and caring enough to find out about results.

Confronting Issues

Some leaders prefer to bury themselves and become invisible to staff, particularly when things are not going well. This type of response to pressure may set up a series of events that will weaken communication throughout the organization. The leader's absence only feeds the rumor mill and leads to unhealthy speculation about the severity of the suspected problem. Thus a minor cutback in staff can quickly get blown up into an impending disaster if staff are forced to rely on rumors for information. By withdrawing to avoid confrontation or bad news, the leader upsets the organization's equilibrium, to which the leader usually contributes by encouraging high staff morale and motivation.

Staff members need to see even more of their leader when things seem to be going astray. Although it sometimes takes extra effort to put oneself at risk by facing a critical issue rather than hoping it will resolve itself, leaders who embrace their role realize that their moods are influential and that their ability to constructively confront issues affecting their staff is as important to their employees' confidence as it is to daily operations. Sheltering or removing oneself from difficult situations sets an example that will only serve to confuse staff at all levels. (Chapter 6 provides some specific suggestions for handling confrontations.)

Embattled executives sometimes also try to back away from needed confrontations by subtly transferring responsibility to others. However, leaders with integrity know that staff members should not have to take the heat for tough decisions and that the executive team should be out in front in the decision-making process. At the same time, leaders must know the value of personal courage and must reward the willingness of staff members to identify their own responsibility in making decisions.

Controlling Energy Flow

Individuals with flagging energy may be unable to cope with rapid change. The health care leader needs to monitor staff energy levels and to know how to provide staff with the renewal they need to respond to the constant changes and challenges in the health care setting. Telephone calls that are not answered in a timely fashion and memos that disappear into the system without response are often symptomatic of declining energy. But the best way for leaders to find out how much energy staff members have for their work is simply to walk around and talk with them.

The leader can do much to help individuals cope under stress. Permitting and even encouraging individuals to take time off helps take the pressure off and provides them with the opportunity to replenish their energy. (Of course, this also applies to the CEO.) Some people (particularly so-called Type A personalities) need encouragement from their supervisor to make taking time off permissible.

Another approach that may help to relieve pressure is to make sure the stressed individual has opportunities for continuing education as a means of gaining a little distance from day-to-day problems. The opportunity to link up with and acquire new knowledge from colleagues often helps individuals to realize that others share their concerns and pressure. Putting things in perspective can be a refreshing and helpful experience.

The leader can also help by setting an "image standard" for the organization (bearing in mind, of course, that different executives have different styles). Despite the assumption that managers come equipped with the ability to effectively organize their own work, just as they do the work of others, many executives need help with controlling the organization and flow of work in their own offices. A messy desk may mean that the individual is busy, but on the other hand, it might suggest that the paperwork has gotten out of hand. Some guidance will not only help prevent burn-out, it will also help the leader monitor and control the crucial flow of energy in the organization.

When a leader senses that a member of the team is becoming overstressed, personal contact with the individual becomes very important. You cannot know the cause of the stress without enough contact to diagnose the problem. Some stressed executives try to conceal the fact that they are "close to the edge" to try to prevent any perception of weakness. In fact, sometimes one of the symptoms of stress is that the individual will try to become invisible to the leader, often canceling scheduled appointments and avoiding other routine contacts. In these situations, it is all the more important for the leader to spend sufficient time with the individual. The first step is to work to reestablish contact and gently probe to find out how things are going. Then, when the relationship is reasonably healthy, the causes of the stress will surface and programs can be designed to help the individual work through the problems.

Along with helping individuals cope with stress, the leader must expect a minimum standard of performance of all staff and should be able to recognize when a staff member's low level of energy can no longer be attributed to the demands of the job. It is not always easy to know how much to bend to individuals' needs, but leaders who are clear about the level of performance they expect, both for themselves and for their staff, will set the best example. If the usual measures fail to renew the individual's energy, the leader will need to probe further to discover the reason for the staff member's declining performance.

In addition to controlling the energy throughout the organization, leaders need to monitor their own energy and commitments as well. For example, those of us who have worked in the health care field for a number of years know that we have an obligation to represent the organization well within the community. Fulfilling community responsibilities requires the ability to balance time and energy, and an awareness that our contributions to the community earn support for the health care organization. Involvement in community affairs also provides many personal benefits to the health care leader, often leading to deepened convictions about the worth of community service. These days organizational pressures make it more difficult for the leader to commit time outside the institution. But failure to keep the organization in the mainstream of the community deprives the organization of needed community support. The stronger the inside team, the easier it is for the CEO to function at the community service level.

Monitoring energy levels also means saving enough energy for non-work-related activities. This is particularly challenging for today's health care executives, who find an unlimited number of demands on their time and feel compelled to respond to as many demands as possible. Individuals who do not reserve energy for themselves and their outside relationships are undertaking a risk not only to themselves and people who are important to them but also to their organization. A leader's home life has as much influence on his or her professional life as does the organizational environment.[1]

As executives take on additional responsibilities, they must be sure that the corporate ladder they are climbing is supported by a solid structure at home. Leaders should keep family members informed of demands on their schedules and help them anticipate business trips and meetings. It is also important to save time for weekday or weekend activities with the family. Although this sounds like common sense (and common courtesy), it is surprising how the demands of the job can deprive executives of a balanced perspective on work and home activities. Leaders who regularly forget to give family members their schedule, or who feel they do not have enough energy or time for their family and friends, should probably consider whether they are devoting too much energy to work. There are few things sadder than to see executives reach the peak of their career only to find that they are alone because they have failed to maintain a balance between personal time and professional time. The demands on the health care leader are undeniably immense, but they should not be the cause of a leader's inability to enjoy a productive and positive personal life.

Learning as a Lifelong Process

Perhaps the single most important factor contributing to an individual's leadership development is commitment to a lifelong process of learning. Excellent leaders make a career out of surpassing barriers that inhibit organizational receptiveness to new knowledge. They seek out the means to use facts and information to produce something useful for the organization. The result may be a better way of doing something, an expanded program, or a new solution to an old problem.

Leaders read. They read books and journals to keep abreast of the changes in their field and the opinions of their colleagues. But perhaps more important is their interest in reading people. Because the best leaders are attentive to the needs of their followers, they are able to apply the tools of management with sensitivity and purpose, adjusting their practices when necessary to meet current conditions and needs.

Too frequently the thirst for new knowledge is dulled by the hectic pace associated with the machinery of bureaucracy. We feel this particularly acutely in health care, with so much pressure from patients, government, and other payers about the escalating costs of care. Leaders sometimes become so immersed in day-to-day events that they fail to appreciate the need to look at career development as a long-term venture. But it is important to recognize that our constant activity must be balanced and fueled by new insights, new information, and new experiences.

It is more than a little disturbing to observe young executives who have much to contribute to health services but who fail to understand the need to invest in their own growth. Those of us who have learned this for ourselves—some of us the hard way—need to help a new generation of leaders stay focused on the essential role that learning plays in building leadership skills. A lifelong commitment to learning requires reading and thinking, and the application of new knowledge to current and changing situations.

Maintaining Optimism and a Sense of Humor

Excellent leaders cultivate optimism even when confronted with potential failure. They do so in part because they recognize that others depend on them to set the mood for the organization as a whole. Although it sometimes seems that there are not a lot of things to be positive about, particularly in health care, the leader's job is to balance every setback with a step forward, to find the positive side of every negative situation. Physicians who encounter life-or-death situations on a regular basis, yet remain optimistic and upbeat as they approach each new patient, show the kind of resilience that should inspire their colleagues in administration.[2]

The leader who has a sense of humor will find it much easier to be hopeful in the face of disheartening circumstances. Humor is extremely important to your own health and to the health of those around you. This is not to suggest that executives should be jokers, nor that they should rely on humor as a means of stroking their own egos or attacking or demeaning colleagues. Rather, it is the ability to appreciate the irony in a situation, or to enjoy the normal give-and-take that occurs between people who like to work together, that will contribute to the leader's optimistic outlook and demeanor.

Protecting Corporate Culture

The health care leader serves as a protector of the organization's corporate culture—all the values, traditions, and history that make up the organizational environment. A strong and vital corporate culture, in which goals and objectives are met because people are engaged in a common effort, provides structure in times of turmoil, financial setbacks, or significant leadership changes. Leaders who understand this should exemplify the desired attitudes and maintain the commitments that are embodied in the corporate culture, and cultivate those attitudes and actions in their staff teams as well. Employees and managers look to senior executives for direction and reinforcement. Although this extremely visible position may be uncomfortable for executives who do not wish to have their actions interpreted as reflective of the organization's goals or interests, it is important to realize that any actions or attitudes expressed by senior executives will contribute to the prevailing culture. Those who lead well accept the important influence they have and cultivate a posture that is consistent with the organization's goals and mission.

Building a Team Effort

The health care leader sometimes functions as a facilitator, drawing team members toward common goals while also encouraging team members to express independent opinions. Finding a balance between helping staff to express ideas and asserting one's own ideas and wishes is one of leadership's greatest challenges, particularly to executives who truly appreciate their staff members and value the concept of teamwork.

Differences of opinion should be expressed in a way that reinforces team integrity. There is a difference between a professional disagreement concerning a problem or project, and an opinion expressed in purely personal terms to attack or degrade another member of the team. Opinions expressed at the personal expense of others cannot be tolerated, and leaders who sense that a discussion is taking a turn in this direction should address it immediately, regardless of any reluctance they may feel to get involved in interactions between staff members.

At the same time as the leader monitors the individual input of staff members, he or she must also be aware of the powerful influence of any dominant personality, including the leader's own, on the orientation of the team. The leader cannot afford to let team members function in a "group think" process in which everyone suppresses their own opinion and acquiesces to a single, strong spokesperson. Powerful leaders need to make sure that opportunities for honest dissension are provided often and with sincerity.

So the leader directs team members toward a common goal. Along the way, he or she provides opportunities for team members to grow, both individually and as a group. Encouraging growth means building confidence. And building confidence sometimes means allowing things to go wrong and taking the responsibility for them when they do. The leader who recognizes the importance of team growth will see that any contribution to the team is ultimately a step toward improving the organization as a whole. Permitting occasional failures is important because individuals learn as much or more from failures as they do from successes. The manager who installs a new laboratory reporting system and then discovers that it is not working for her staff will learn much more by working with and being supported by the staff during the partial failure than she would if the failure were considered a calamity that could threaten her job. If staff members are bound by the expectation that failure is unacceptable, tension levels will rise and the organization will lose its capacity for innovation. The inability to accept the possibility of failure will come home to haunt the leader because members of the team will begin to refuse to step forward to resolve problems and issues, since they perceive that by doing so they will jeopardize their positions.

Conclusion

By definition, the leader is "out front," setting examples and demonstrating a high order of commitment to achieving both personal and organizational goals. The true leader understands the obligations and responsibilities that come along with the leadership role and is willing to accept the challenges. Serving the interests of the organization with a sense of personal and professional integrity means looking closely and honestly at your own values and commitments. One's personal interests might not always seem consistent with the organization's stated or unstated needs. At those times, leaders must either challenge themselves to fulfill their professional obligations without compromising personal standards, or they must change their standards to meet those espoused by the organization.

Notes

1. J. Meston, "If It Gets Sloppy Eat It Over the Sink," *Executive Excellence* 5, no. 10 (1986): 4.
2. W. Bennis and B. Namus, *Leaders: The Strategies for Taking Charge* (New York: Harper & Row, 1984).

PART II

DIRECTION: LEADING THE TEAM

4

BUILDING THE HEALTH CARE
MANAGEMENT TEAM

Case in Point

At a professional meeting several years ago, a group of us were sitting around exchanging "war stories," when a good friend of mine related an interesting experience about his efforts to make a team player out of an overly aggressive manager.

My friend was at the helm as the administrator of a large group practice. One of his senior associate administrators was an effective operator who had learned in his previous position in a large hospital that the best way to get things done was to use power to bring about solutions. He found that by being pushy he could "bulldoze" decisions through the system and no one would stop him. Under his direction, things happened and goals were met, but not without a significant cost to the staff's team spirit.

Colleagues learned that direct confrontation with the associate was painful and unproductive, so they looked for creative ways to avoid inter-action. Since the associate's budgets were on target, his poor interpersonal skills were tolerated by the administration. However, a lawsuit filed by a for-mer employee who claimed discrimination (and the subsequent out-of-court settlement of the claim) added fuel to the fire.

My friend the CEO simply did not recognize the detrimental effect this had on the staff. Everyone probably wondered why he tolerated a situation that was so demoralizing, but because they did not share their perception of the problem, it took a long time for him to find out how bad things were. In retrospect, he said, he realized that he was probably being shielded from the seriousness of the situation because of his close relationship with the associate (which was common knowledge among the staff).

Complaints began to accelerate and my friend finally realized that he had only been seeing the tip of the iceberg. He had been shielded from nearly all of the bad news and had accepted operational results as evidence of the associate's competence. He had accepted some poor interpersonal behavior on the premise that tough decisions had to be made and, as he himself often said, "you can't please everyone." But finally it was time to act.

A series of one-on-one meetings was set up. At the first meeting, my friend pulled no punches. He related his discovery that people were being trampled and told the associate that his behavior was out of line with the culture of the organization. The associate would simply have to adjust his behavior or prepare to leave.

It was a devastating experience for the associate, but it was not just a one-sided conversation. My friend listened carefully as his associate explained that he thought that he was expected to get results and did not realize that teamwork was so high on the organization's list of values and expectations.

Then an interesting event took place. In the second meeting, the associate related that he had been doing some real soul-searching. He liked his work and wanted to succeed. The associate went on to say that in his entire career no one had ever really laid it out as my friend had done. No one had given him an honest appraisal of negative aspects of his performance.

As time went on, it became apparent that things were improving. The associate began to change his behavior and became much more cooperative. My friend said he took great care to give feedback to his associate to reinforce the change in behavior and to try to emphasize the importance of team interaction. When it was time to plan for the traditional spring management potluck dinner, the associate volunteered to organize the event—an action that was totally unexpected and out of character with the individual's previous performance. Obviously wounds were healing, and while the associate's approach still tended to "power through" decisions, much progress had been made toward a more cooperative, team-oriented management style.

In any health care organization, creativity and innovation are enhanced by a strong management team. Team building is the ultimate in administrative orchestration—it requires discipline, balance, and hard work. Health care executives who want to lead their organizations into the twenty-first century will need to acquire team-building skills and to use their teams to respond to the continuing changes ahead.

Building effective teams is especially difficult in the health care setting. Medical organizations are both hierarchical in structure and staffed with specialists, many of whom relate more closely to their specialty than to the organization as a whole. Physicians, nurses, and pharmacists, for example, tend to build relationships within the clinical environment rather than becoming part of organizational relationships. Thus the health care leader has a particularly difficult task and must rely heavily on the support of an effective management team to support teamwork throughout the organization.

Challenging Traditional Management Practices

The health care organizations that are best positioned for the future are those in which leaders stimulate organizational flexibility, and focus on multidisciplinary teams as the means to make good decisions. Health care leaders who are interested in team building in the 1990s must modify traditional practices that are based on control from the top. They must learn more about change and renewal, and must constantly be on guard against the development of self-serving bureaucracies that counteract the synergism of effective team operation.

Perhaps the first step toward creating a functional management team is to reevaluate the existing management structure. Traditional habits need to be challenged, and decision-making processes need to be streamlined. Once the team functions effectively, it will be linked with other staff teams, so the leader must work hard to eliminate any barriers to flexibility and creativity.

In *The Renewal Factor*, Robert Waterman reports on how the country's "best" companies maintain their competitive edge. He advocates some change for change's sake, noting that leaders in competitive companies create change processes in order to develop an enterprising attitude.[1] These leaders treat all employees as potential sources of creative input. Pushing decision making down into the organization is what change through empowerment is all about.

Simplifying the organizational structure (with more people reporting to fewer) is in itself a process that aids team building. Executives who have more people reporting to them must learn to be more trusting of the judgment of their staff or they will flounder under the weight of detail. Many organizations are surprised at how well a simplified structure works. For example, several years ago, the Union Pacific Railroad Company took drastic steps in this regard. The company eliminated an entire layer of management (some 600 positions) and discovered that the effective executive was capable of overseeing many more individuals than management theorists previously thought possible.

This kind of structural simplification has many possible implications for the health care field. The subspecialization and fragmentation of so many occupations in health services has led to the creation of very complex reporting relationships. But the hospital or group practice of the future will find that cross-training to streamline managerial responsibilities will be essential for maintaining financial and service viability. Who is to say that a highly competent laboratory manager is incapable of also managing other departments, unless someone gives it a try? (A further discussion of the process of streamlining the organization can be found in Chapter 12.)

Selecting the Management Team

The leader should begin the process of identifying potential new members for the management team by doing an assessment of the strengths and weaknesses of the existing staff in relation to the needs and goals of the organization. Members of the management team should be ranked according to their abilities in four areas:

1. *Technical competence.* Are the managers competent to perform their particular specialty, and are their skills and knowledge up-to-date?

2. *Interpersonal skills.* Do the potential team members care about fellow employees and take the time to know and understand what it is that makes a team function (trust, professional respect, and so on)? Are members of the team recognized as leaders, and how is this demonstrated? Are these leaders fair and capable of confronting and resolving people problems?

3. *Ability to identify and solve problems.* Can they address problems from both a tactical and a strategic angle? Are alternatives adequately inventoried and is the potential impact of decisions on the organization identified and a part of recommended solutions? Or do team members successfully identify a problem but then simply transfer the problem to another (i.e., moving monkeys from one person's back to another's)?

4. *Leadership ability.* Are the team members really capable of leading others? Are they capable of communicating ideas and then energizing those around them in order to achieve a specific goal? Team members might be geniuses in a technical sense, but if they cannot lead and communicate ideas in the process the organization will not be fully served.

Balance: Rounding Out the Team

The leader must also examine the balance of skills on the management team. If the existing team lacks competency in a particular area—for example, financial affairs—then it may be necessary to strengthen the team by adding an individual with this skill or by providing existing members with special training. If the senior executive needs to devote substantial time to outside activities (such as community or professional engagements), it is essential that strong operational professionals are in place to conduct and direct internal affairs.

When leaders new to an organization inherit existing teams, they have the special challenge of merging their personal style with the existing team while simultaneously assessing and adjusting assignments. A special look at team balance is important in this situation since the incoming executive usually arrives with different strengths and weaknesses than the previous leader had.

Because it takes such a long time to build a team, any change in the team's composition should be conducted very carefully. Teams seem to be easy to destroy but difficult to build. Organizations that have had frequent changes in leadership learn this lesson the hard way as they try to carry on in a constant state of flux.

Involving Physicians in Management

Although the typical organizational structure in the 1970s and 1980s separated functions of the governing board from those of the medical staff and management, this concept is now as obsolete as the three-legged milking stool. Today's environment requires efficient, effective, and integrated teams drawing on all essential professional disciplines (not just physicians but nurses and others as well). Physicians need to be key participants in decision making in today's health care organizations, and organizations need to identify and involve physicians who have the interest, instincts, and competence to help manage and lead.

The first step in developing a management orientation that includes physicians is to work on dispelling stereotypes and narrow attitudes held by both administrators and physicians. Some health care executives continue to believe that physician involvement in management would be detrimental to the health care organization. Perhaps some administrators, particularly those have had difficult confrontations with physicians, view physician involvement as personally threatening. This is a normal reaction to a perceived threat, but it is an attitude that administrators cannot afford to have in this era.

Although a growing number of physicians are intrigued with administrative processes, too much association with management is often perceived by other medical staff members as a sign of clinical disinterest (or incompetence). In addition, many physicians seem to be conditioned, beginning with their clinical schooling, to consider administrators as bureaucrats. This attitude may be partly responsible for the push by physician organizations to "take back management from lay administration." Younger administrators and physicians seem to face fewer of these traditional attitude problems, but there are still a considerable number in both camps who would prefer to remain separate. These attitudes are unfortunate; they will lead only to further fragmentation within the health care system. Building administrator-physician teams requires that an organizational attitude be fostered that supports physician involvement in decision making. The attitude must start at the top of the organization. Once this commitment is accepted as a part of the organization's culture, then the other steps will flow more naturally.

In team building with physicians, health care executives should consider adopting a "buddy system" to link physicians and administrators on projects, to encourage involvement, and to reward cooperation that results in the integration of professional and management disciplines. When professional administrators and physicians work together, they gain both respect for their different orientations and skills, and the satisfaction of sharing and achieving a common goal.

Physician participation in administration must be based on more than an expressed interest. Leaders in the organization need to evaluate physicians on their administrative skills, not just their clinical ability. Techniques used in evaluating nonphysician administrators work just as well to evaluate the administrative skills of the physician.

For a joint administrator-physician team to be effective, there must be interpersonal respect, credibility, and compatibility. As noted earlier, teams function best when members recognize that others on the team have skills that complement their own. So team balance, aided by clear definition of roles, is essential. Role definition enhances collaboration and minimizes competition between team members by clarifying levels of power and authority. On the other hand, too much definition creates barriers to effective team operation by over-compartmentalizing functions. Adequately rewarding team members who function as team players contributes to the process of integrating different skills and disciplines and applying them to a common cause. Executives can build the credibility of administrator-physician teams by looking for ways to credit program or project outcomes to the total team.

Management should also recognize the need for continuing management education for both physicians and other administrators involved in teams. A physician is not necessarily qualified to manage administrative affairs simply by virtue of a degree in medicine. Physicians who assume positions of management responsibility may feel vulnerable, although they may also be unwilling to admit to a lack of management knowledge. Organizations should provide continuing education opportunities for physicians to enhance their administrative skills. Physicians who are new to management can benefit from the knowledge of experienced administrators (both physicians and nonphysicians), so leaders might consider sending teams of administrators and physicians together to these continuing education conferences.

Some organizations seem to be marketing programs exclusively for physicians with the subtle message that physicians should leave the administrator behind and learn what management is really all about. One of the worst things that an executive can do, after deliberately creating administrator-physician teams, is to support or even tolerate this "us versus them" attitude. The leader is in the best position to stop this attitude once it has started and to build in its stead a more positive, cooperative atmosphere.

Cultivating the Team Spirit

Organizations that are growing, and that are creative and innovative, are able to grow because of management continuity and stability. Even under excellent leadership, it can take three to five years of solid work and involvement for a group of individuals to complete the process of building an effective team. When management experts suggest to younger colleagues that they should relocate to another organization every three years or so if they want to advance in their careers, their advice does a disservice to both the organization and to the individual staff members. Too much movement deprives younger professionals of the experience of a full cycle of team development.

Positive Team Dynamics

A team must be more than a collection of individuals. A functioning team is a cohesive, interdependent, and focused group that knows where it is going. All members should participate in setting team goals. Team members are able to clearly articulate objectives that relate to the mission of the organization. The leader will want to create an environment in which the following dynamics can occur within the team:

1. The team and its members recognize that the overall mission of the organization is more important than personal ambition.
2. There is a high level of interpersonal confidence and trust, which allows team members to cross traditional organizational lines. Turf issues are minimized and managers share information with each

other in a common cause. The director of patient services, for example, would feel free to alert the chief financial officer well in advance of month-end reports if departmental budget variations resulted from variations in caseload.

3. The team members sense that personal and professional security are, in fact, interdependent.

4. There is a high level of organizational intimacy. Team members exchange information openly and are aware of the problems and frustrations faced by their colleagues.

5. Team members possess enough self-confidence to disagree with each other and to debate issues from different viewpoints. But once a decision is made the team rallies and closes ranks to move programs forward with enthusiasm.

6. Team members identify with team success. They are willing to share the limelight and are diligent about sharing credit for successes with their colleagues. (One interesting check to determine how much team members value the team is to scan memos written by leaders and team members. If the memos are sprinkled with many references to self (I) rather than with references to team activity (we), the organization may need some work on the team-building process.)

Leaders also recognize that there will be times when teams experience conflict. Leaders must be prepared to confront individuals who play politics, guard turf, fail to exchange information, or engage in other destructive actions. Leaders must also be supportive of individuals on the team who disagree on the proper solution to problems, but they should insist that such disagreements be carried out on a professional basis, not through personal attacks or infighting.

The Leadership Role

Maintaining a team over time demands constant attention. When an effective team is in place, it is a pure delight for the experienced leader. The ultimate effective team is a group of individuals who balance each other, possess interdependency based on mutual respect, and believe that the outcome of the team effort is worth more than the contributions of any single member of the team. Constant surveillance—to fine-tune the team's work and to make sure that the team's expectations are being met—is what produces dynamic and on-target results. The leader's role as "monitor" raises two obvious concerns—how closely to participate, and what the team's expectations will be.

Distance. Every team leader faces the question of how close to get, both personally and professionally, to team members. Distance provides objectivity, but closeness encourages the loyalty and friendship that are essential to fueling the team's desire to engage totally in a common effort. Is it even possible that too much familiarity may create problems when it comes time to resolve conflict or confront difficult situations? Is the team leader subject to criticism for collaborating more closely with some team members than with others?

Too much personal closeness can bias judgment. Leaders who fail to recognize this can easily develop a team whose work revolves almost entirely around the leader's personality (a leadership cult). Sometimes even strong, competent leaders inadvertently surround themselves with individuals who quietly reinforce their leader's ego. Team members gradually become subservient, and the leader just as gradually begins to accumulate excessive power. The leader does not need to be detached or cold, but some distance may help in maintaining the right perspective when counseling team members or interceding to develop a common direction.

What should the staff expect? Team members should have high expectations for their leader. Executives who genuinely espouse a high standard for their own performance will want team members who challenge them to meet that standard. In particular, teams need leaders who are able to do the following:

1. *Be consistent.* The executive who is unpredictable and moody makes it difficult for team members to produce good results, and in the end a lack of consistency in temperament inevitably curtails communication and organizational effectiveness.

2. *Value their team members' skills and judgment.* Senior executives should spend a sufficient amount of time really listening and receiving input—and not simply talking—so that managers and team members have the opportunity to thoroughly present programs and recommendations.

3. *Delegate.* Team members and managers should expect that projects will be delegated and that the senior executive will not need to direct each activity. Too much supervision kills individual initiative.

4. *Provide overall direction.* The leader's role is to establish and monitor organizational goals and objectives. Much of the detail and content of strategies leading to attainment of these objectives should be delegated to others.

5. *Share the spotlight.* Team members should be able to count on the executive to give the credit for particular successes to the appropriate staff member. In addition, they should be able to trust that

they will be informed of decisions and the rationale behind them. If senior executives are able to rely on facts and information received from middle managers and others, they in turn should share their thoughts with their colleagues.

Working with the Team

Health care executives and their management teams will be expected to lead health care organizations through the industry's rough waters in the years ahead. The health care leader's survival depends on being able to count on team members to establish priorities, handle long-term assignments, and report on the process and progress of these assignments in a timely fashion. If one team member fails to produce, others may be required to backtrack, and organizational gains may be delayed or deferred. Thus all members of the team have to be capable of looking beyond the most immediate next step in the process.

Expectations for Team Behavior

As the leader of the management team, you want people who can meet a number of basic expectations. First, you want team members to be diligent about follow-up. Being able to rely on team members means knowing that they will follow through on assignments. Nothing is more disappointing than expecting a team member to handle a project and discovering that the responsibility has been ignored. If, for example, you have asked a project leader to keep the medical staff fully informed on the development of a hospital–medical staff joint venture, and the project leader fails to do so, it will be difficult to continue with the same confidence in the project leader's credibility. Management team members should know this better than anyone, since follow-up is the bread and butter of daily management. Even beyond the need to get the job done, interpersonal relationships depend on trust levels between members of the team regarding each individual's timely contribution to the team's goal. If a project cannot be completed for reasons beyond the individual's control, that individual has a responsibility to keep abreast of the situation rather than allowing the project to slide.

Second, when a team member needs to consult with a senior executive, the executive should ask for the information to be reported in a summary fashion and not in exorbitant detail. Team members should be encouraged to cultivate a sense of the appropriate degree of detail required to present a particular subject. If the particular project has higher risks for the organization, more detail may well be required. On the other hand, a staff member who feels compelled to explain every detail of the rationale for every decision is simply wasting time, especially if the leader is only interested in the overall status of the project. It is the team leader's responsibility to spell out the level of detail needed, and it is often most helpful to ask team members to report exceptional situations rather than routine matters.

If a team member consistently overreports, the executive might be wise to question the team member's motivation and should make clear what is expected. Is the team member relating so much detail because of a lack of confidence in the conclusion? Or is the team member just testing ideas and reactions before arriving at a conclusion? (This may be necessary in many cases to obtain a sense of direction, but it is not a process that should be followed routinely.) The executive should consider whether the team member is providing a lot of detail as a means of avoiding making a decision or recommendation.

The executive also relies on members of the management team to express their thoughts in writing. If team members are unable to organize material adequately in writing, senior executives should suspect that the program or issue at hand may not be worked out sufficiently. A CEO might make a brilliant verbal presentation to the hospital board about a new outreach program, but the inability to express this enthusiasm in writing could result in the project's failure if the project needs to be backed up by written communication from the staff. Staff members may find it easier to discuss ideas than to take the time and effort required to organize them thoughtfully and put them down in writing. This is not to suggest that opportunities for the oral exchange of ideas should be avoided, nor is it a suggestion that good paperwork is an adequate substitute for a good oral presentation. But if a proposal under consideration carries high risks and involves a significant organizational policy or program, it is reasonable to expect that those responsible for submitting the ideas can provide conclusions and summaries, both in oral presentations and in writing.

Third, team members should be capable of self-discipline, particularly with regard to adherence to timelines and schedules. Answering mail (and telephone calls) promptly represents good organizational hygiene. Team members need to understand that their colleagues in other hospitals and organizations are busy too, and that a rapid and concise process of moving information back and forth is crucial if activities are to move forward successfully. Effective executives generally advocate "concise request" and "prompt response" policies, which recognize that too many programs are ineffectively implemented because someone did not follow through.

Team members' performance is measured to a considerable degree by their ability to honor commitments. The process of building personal credibility by turning information around is extremely important. Executives who apply high standards to their management team in this regard must apply them equally to themselves.

Fourth, team members should be willing and able to share information with the rest of the team and with the senior executive to aid in informed decision making. Health care executives frequently find themselves in difficult positions with respect to making complicated decisions, especially when resources are limited. How should the CEO decide whether to commit to a program replacing outdated surgical suites or to invest in building a medical office building adjacent to the hospital? Wise executive leaders understand that they will not be right all the time; they deal with operating based on a percentage of error. But although the executive may not be overly endowed with knowledge on the internal operations of a particular department, he or she has to develop an effective means of evaluating the performance of the unit as a whole. Senior executives should encourage and expect team members to share appropriate information both with each other and with their leader.

Finally, the leader needs team members to be willing and able to support decisions. The leader should expect that open debate and exchange of thoughts about projects or policy matters will occur at all levels in the organization, but particularly among management team members. Once decisions have been made, there should be a general expectation that the members of the team, while being encouraged to express private opinions to senior executives and other team members, should not publicly display their disagreement with any new policy. Nothing is gained, for example, when a decision is made to reduce employee overtime pay by requiring that all overtime be authorized by a supervisor, if half the management staff reluctantly communicates the new policy to their employees as if they had no part in the decision-making process. Once a key decision has been made, the senior executive should legitimately expect that members of the team will function as an integrated unit and not as a group of individual dissenters.

Delegating in Troubled Times

Traditional wisdom suggests that the larger an organization is, the greater the number of responsibilities that should be delegated out of the leader's office. Trust your subordinates, we hear, and do not overmanage. Although this is generally wise advice, it works best in an era of tranquility and predictability—which this certainly is not. The real test of a leader's ability to delegate takes place in times of organizational stress and turmoil, when the temptation to oversee (translate: interfere) surfaces in nearly every health care executive.

The amount of leeway provided subordinates is proportionately related to the amount of turmoil the organization is experiencing. In times of stability and predictability, the senior executive should delegate as much as possible. This is a way to give subordinates opportunities to learn without great risk to the organization. But when the environment changes and the stress factor builds, the senior executive must probe deeper to increase the amount and quality of feedback, and to ensure that operating decisions are on track.

The process of increasing intervention affects managers at all levels of the organization. After periods of quasi-independence, the invasion of a senior executive who begins to question what is going on will usually be viewed as an indication of mistrust. A senior executive with a strong team, who delegates responsibility and then suddenly begins to query subordinates on operational issues, sends mixed messages to staff.

A change in style and practice raises questions, and concern is heightened if the senior executive suddenly gets more involved in decision making at lower levels in the organization. One of the first steps for the senior executive to take, if circumstances warrant intervention, is to tell team members why more information is needed now than was needed earlier. It is important for the team to anticipate the need to better inform the CEO when organizational conditions veer from the norm.

The CEO's responsibility is to communicate priorities and needs during a volatile time period and to prepare the management team to accept such changes in direction without loss of trust.[2] Team members should be made aware that the CEO may have to make decisions without consulting with all parties, particularly in a crisis situation. Discipline and acceptance of authority is required at such times. However, the CEO should also explain the parameters of the action and the reasons for having to intercede. It is then up to the manager to adapt to this new (and, it is hoped, temporary) strategic approach.

Under conditions of unusual stress, leaders will do well to adhere to a few basic principles with regard to delegation:

1. The more you can rely on your management team's judgment (not just competency), the more you can delegate to them. If they are able to consistently anticipate your need to know, they are obviously demonstrating evidence of good judgment.

2. If the team has consistently accomplished assignments and met previous commitments, it will be easier to delegate additional assignments to them when the going gets rough. This does not mean that the CEO should eliminate usual and customary follow-up mechanisms but simply that follow-up monitoring can be eased. An

experienced team, which has proven its credibility, can be relied upon to handle added assignments in periods of stress.

3. During times of organizational stress, the CEO should not be timid about increasing requests for information but should be careful to communicate why the information is needed. Teamwork is undermined by keeping team members in the dark. Sharing concerns, without divulging privileged information, will build the trust you need to make it through the crisis.

4. When delegating, delegate clearly and effectively. Avoid giving the team an assignment one day and pulling it away the next. Set time frames that are realistic, and enlist the team's participation in setting the deadlines. If more than one staff team will be involved in a project, make sure that managers know their respective assignments. Complicated assignments should be conveyed both verbally and in writing to minimize misunderstandings.

5. Make sure the team gets clear closure when the assignment and the immediate crisis is over. Avoid leaving loose strings hanging in the organization. The administration of health services is so complicated that everything that can be done to provide clean, clear fields of action, uncluttered by half-completed projects or partially fulfilled objectives, will aid in creating and nurturing an effective, efficient organization.

Successful delegation is the oil that lubricates decision making, but delegation does not relieve the leader of overall accountability. The way a leader delegates is, of course, dependent upon the competence and experience of team members. Every assignment delegated probably touches on another project or program, so careful coordination is essential. The executive is responsible for making sure that, even under the most stressful conditions, the management team is able to operate with a sense of direction.

Creativity and Teamwork

Since no one person in an organization controls the organization's potential for creativity, it is useful to reflect on how to recognize and nurture creativity in team members. In the hospital or the medical group practice setting, creativity can be obscured or constrained by the organizational environment. Competition or confusion in direction can also make it more difficult for individuals to be creative. For example, when physicians in a medical group practice disagree with each other about a specific decision, their creative energy may be used up just by trying to keep the peace. The leader should learn to recognize those who are creatively inclined and to make it possible for such individuals to prosper. The first step in that direction is to look at individual performance and end results, instead of focusing on personality or level of conformance.

Recognizing Creative Characteristics

In every organization, there are some who not only perform very competently in their assigned tasks but who also reach out and touch others in the organization. The creative person blossoms when confronted with the unusual and seems to be intrigued with process. The creative person frequently displays natural enthusiasm, self-confidence, reflective qualities, and a certain appreciation for detail. He or she is willing to speak up and take risks, possesses good communication skills, and displays a high degree of personal integrity.

Creative individuals seem to be driven to shape change. They may not always know exactly where they are going, but they resist the status quo. Because they are often looking to make things better, they are an invaluable resource for the organization, which can only be creative if it values the creative input of individuals within the structure.

Fostering Creativity

There may be individuals on your management team who, because they fear change and prefer the status quo, will go to considerable lengths to derail creative people around them. Others may resent a creative member of the team who enjoys the challenges that the team has before it. Creative people often are able to find humor in even the most bizarre situations, which allows them to maintain a mental balance and perspective in all that they do at work and at home. To encourage all team members to call on their own creative abilities, it is important to develop a style of working with the team that will generate and reward innovation and creative attitudes.

The management styles that are best suited for developing innovation and creativity within the management team are those that (1) encourage the easy flow of information between managers, physicians, and employees, and therefore result in trusting relationships and collaborative decision-making practices; (2) perpetuate a unified sense of purpose (particularly regarding patient care) through succeeding generations of medical and administrative leaders; (3) emphasize the dignity of the individual employee and the value of his or her potential contribution; and (4) foster positive and supportive attitudes to create a sense of excitement that can be transferred and conveyed vertically and horizontally within the organization. These are crucial ingredients in the vital, dynamic health services setting.

Recognizing the Value of Human Resources

To stimulate creativity, many leaders seek ways to flatten the organizational structure to provide management team members with more professional opportunities. They find they are able both to accomplish more with less and to meet organizational objectives and goals more effectively. But in the process of attaining these worthwhile goals, some executives develop a blind spot. They have rewarded the intellectual and professional abilities of their managers and have neglected staff members whose creativity is equally valuable to the organization but who are several steps removed from day-to-day contact with the senior executive.

The untapped wealth that can really make a difference in preserving and enhancing quality and service in most health care organizations lies not in the executive's corporate office but instead in the supervisor's office, at the patient's bedside, or in the support systems departments. It is a major event, almost a revelation, when an executive who is used to a top-down bureaucratic style of management discovers the insight of employees who work at a distance from the head office.

Some time ago, a large health services organization was experiencing considerable growth. The CEO recognized that there was a growing communication problem between the medical staff and the corporate structure. Traditional methods of communication that worked in the past when the organization was smaller simply were no longer doing the job. In addition, restructuring had occurred and the culture had changed. Physicians previously were located on site but now were involved in a number of satellite sites as well. Communications could no longer be handled on a one-on-one basis.

A typical administrative approach might have been to convene a carefully selected task force, including physicians and others, to consider the communication dilemma. The less conventional approach used by the CEO in this case was to assemble the members of the public relations department, who by the nature of their activity spend considerable time on communication. The public relations group gathered together, the chief executive officer outlined the problem, and the group was asked to conduct a "sky is the limit" brainstorming session. The problem was defined simply as a need to "improve communications with members of our medical staff." The department manager was asked to preside; the CEO only laid out the problem. Challenged by the task and invigorated by being asked to participate in this fashion, the group responded magnificently with a considerable number of initiatives.

The point, of course, is that executives should not think that they are the only experts simply because they are closest to the nerve center of the organization. Contemporary executives who succeed are usually those who learn to recognize that many of their colleagues possess more technical expertise than they do. There are latent and untapped resources in every organization, but it takes a sensitive and wise executive who is willing to risk displaying some lack of expertise to increase the involvement of staff members in creative problem solving.

Evaluating the Team

Traditional methods of evaluating team output focus on measuring achievement of the team's objectives and goals. But performance evaluation should also address the "chemistry" between the team leader and members, as well as the type and frequency of feedback that team members receive. Evaluating their performance in crisis situations and surveying the team during stable times are two of the best ways to measure team effectiveness.

The Team in Crisis: A Measuring Stick

The ultimate test of the team's effectiveness occurs in a crisis (for example, the need to downsize the organization). Can you depend on the team being together, or is it fragmented? In moments of crisis, individuals and organizations respond somewhat predictably. Individuals under attack become much more control oriented, so management styles often change, sending a confusing message to staff. Rather than responding to the crisis by concentrating on their own initiatives, the management team should collaborate to ensure that staff see the virtues of continuing to work together.

Effective leaders are conscious that bad news will always be filtered. They will work diligently to maintain open communication throughout the organization, to offset the possibility of being "blind-sided" because employees fear that the bearer of any bad news will receive the brunt of the leader's criticism. The effective leader also knows that when news flows easily throughout the organization, it is a sign that the management team is healthy.

The Stable Team: Surveying

There are a number of mechanisms available to the leader for monitoring team performance, one of which is to use a carefully designed questionnaire. The team itself can be asked to design the survey instrument to measure how they relate to each other (and how different teams within the same organization relate to each other).

In the example in Exhibit 4.1, 12 senior officials (including the CEO) were listed on the instrument. All members being evaluated were asked to rank each of their 11 colleagues on their competence, the quality of their

Exhibit 4.1 Sample Survey Form

Administrative Team Assessment

Instructions

1. Read the definitions of the criteria and then rate each team member.
2. Do *not* sign form.
3. Return to Administration in a sealed confidential envelope before January 15.
4. Rate each team member on a scale of 1 to 6, with 6 representing excellence.

		Criteria	
Team Members	*Competency*	*Interpersonal Relationships*	*Trust & Value*
George Aubrey	_____	_____	_____
Bill Bond	_____	_____	_____
Jim Borton	_____	_____	_____
Neal Burstrom	_____	_____	_____
Ann Daniels	_____	_____	_____
Inga Hutton	_____	_____	_____
Joy Jensen	_____	_____	_____
Patricia Main	_____	_____	_____
Marion Moores	_____	_____	_____
Dan Olsen	_____	_____	_____
Bob Polk	_____	_____	_____
Michael Rust	_____	_____	_____

Continued

Exhibit 4.1   Continued

Definitions:
Please review these definitions before completing form.

Competency refers to your general perception of how the individual performs in his or her area of responsibility. Are correct decisions made? How is the individual being ranked for his or her competency?

Interpersonal relationships refers to the individual's proficiency as a team participant. Does he or she focus properly on organizational goals and is he or she capable of building esprit de corps with superiors, colleagues, and subordinates?

Trust and value refer to whether the individual is usually perceived as being trustworthy. Will he or she share information willingly? Do you respect the individual's personal and interpersonal values in decision making?

Note: This survey tool is not intended to be a precise measurement of performance; it serves only as a broad measure of perceptions of competency, interpersonal relationships, and terms of trust and value.

---

interpersonal relationships, and their sense of values and ethics. These three factors were intentionally selected to reveal subjective attitudes and perceptions, rather than to measure traditional performance criteria. The survey instrument was distributed with a cover memo stressing that the identity of the individual would be kept confidential but that the chief operating officers of the subsidiary units would each receive a summary of the survey. (Participants were also requested not to sign the survey instrument.)

The cover memorandum also indicated that the administrators would be asked to meet on a one-on-one basis with the chief executive officer. The CEO had reviewed the process with several key staff since it was important that they concur with the process. (If the key subordinates had not wanted to participate, the CEO might have suspected that there was some level of distrust or a problem with communication.)

The final step involved interviews by the corporate CEO with the 12 managers being evaluated. During the interview, three questions were asked. First, "What is your evaluation of the team's performance?" (It was important here that the CEO not raise specific issues or questions that would have suggested a preferred response.)

The second question was, "If you were in charge (of the organization), would you do anything differently?" Again, care was taken to not lead the participant to a particular response. This provided an opportunity for the CEO to get indirect feedback from the team member.

The third question was, "As a CEO, I sometimes have little feedback on my performance. If you were in my position, would you do anything differently?" This question helps focus on specific problems or concerns that are being created by the CEO.

The individuals then were asked to rank the performance of the team on a scale of 1 to 10 (with 10 being high), and in doing so, they were asked to rank the team by comparing them with the organization's competition. (The competition was not defined.) The purpose of the question was to obtain a response to help evaluate overall team effort. This question also provided individuals with the opportunity to complete the interview on a positive note. (Even if there are internal problems, the team usually perceives its collective output as being better than most.) The interview was closed with a reminder of the confidentiality of the process and an expression of appreciation for the participant's candor.

Monitoring team performance is so important that unconventional approaches such as this may be worth considering. The contemporary leader looks for opportunities to test, to try, and to experiment with nontraditional approaches, yet the approaches selected must respect the integrity of the individual and the organizational structure.

Conclusion

Successful health care executives build teams and nourish them constantly. Strong leaders who are willing to modify traditional practices, to learn about change and renewal practices, and to provide opportunities for managers and other staff to take responsibility and make decisions usually foster the most productive team players. The team-building process must be continuous since the addition of even one new member can profoundly change the chemistry of the group. The needs of the organization are also constantly changing. The team leader really functions like the leader of an orchestra, conducting the affairs of the corporation in a fashion that blends and matches the needs of the organization with the talents of the management team. The goal is to accomplish the organizational mission and to create a management team that grows stronger in the process.

Notes

1. R. H. Waterman, Jr., *The Renewal Factor: How the Best Get and Keep the Competitive Edge* (New York: Bantam Books, Inc., 1987).
2. D. S. Ridderheim, "The Anatomy of Change," *Hospital & Health Services Administration* 31, no. 3 (1986): 7–21.

5

Bringing Up the New Team: Orientation through Mentoring

Case in Point

Many years ago, a physician and medical leader in our organization took a special interest in my career. I was a struggling assistant administrator, learning the business and quite possibly in over my head, and Joe would drop by from time to time and give me feedback on how I was doing. I looked up to him both because of his many years of experience and because of his willingness to be candid about the job I was doing. One conversation stands out as if it happened yesterday.

Joe came in and closed the door of my 6-by-9 foot office. After a few pleasantries he got to the point. "I don't think you will make it in this field," he said. I asked him to elaborate. He said that dealing with physicians was a rough business, and he didn't think I would survive because I was not tough enough. I would have to be tougher to make it, he said, and then he left the room.

I was the sole supporter of my young family, so his cautionary words struck home. After overcoming the shock of hearing his piece of advice, I gave it a lot of thought. Rather than scaring me out of the business, he had given me the motivation to work harder. It meant a lot that he had cared enough about my career to risk making me angry, and his comments helped me to prepare myself for the difficult decisions ahead.

One of the keys to successful teamwork is making sure that the team benefits from new influences and insights as new staff are brought into the organization. When new members are added to any team, the health care leader has two major responsibilities: first, to provide the new member with opportunities to learn from and share information with seasoned professionals in the organization, and second, to orient the new member to the organization's values and expectations for behavior and performance. A well-developed mentoring program can address both of these needs, providing direction to both the individual and the team.

The Value of Mentoring

After interviewing 150 executives from Fortune 500 corporations, Michael Zey concluded that a positive mentoring relationship was often the single most important factor contributing to an individual's corporate success, even more important than the much-touted master's degree in business administration.[1]

Mentoring is one of the best ways to build continuing educational experiences, both for young professionals and for established health care managers and executives. The mentor provides fuel for the new employee's enthusiasm, and the new staff member provides fresh insight into problems faced by the more senior, and perhaps more traditional, staff member.

Establishing a Mentoring Program

Who Are the Right Candidates?

The mentoring relationship is often most beneficial for employees who have just finished college degrees. As they move from campus to practice, some new graduates find that they miss the easy access to faculty and the free exchange of thoughts and ideas with peers, which were the hallmarks of their college careers. Once they move into the health care field they lose the security offered by a carefully developed curriculum with defined expectations. Flexibility is the rule in the health care setting, and inexperienced employees may have difficulty adapting to the quickened pace. A new employee must assume increasing responsibility for his or her development. The mentor is in a perfect position to influence the individual's professional development and outcome.

The mentor helps by quietly tracking the individual's experiences on the job to see if they include growth and learning opportunities, and if not, to help guide the individual in seeking such opportunities. A good mentor also monitors the organization to ensure that it accommodates the individual's need to work with others who can share their knowledge and experience. Fundamentally, the mentor is responsible for overseeing—keeping in touch and gently guiding—the individual, but without creating internal conflict or a perception of special privilege.

Similarly, when an individual moves from one health care organization to another, a mentoring relationship can enhance the transfer of knowledge and enrich the professional experience by lending continuity to the process. If trust levels are high between the parties involved, any gaps in experience can be identified early and subsequently filled. As the individual moves on, the mentor should take the opportunity to give closure to the process by providing a thorough and candid appraisal of the individual's performance. This is not the time to overlook deficiencies. Part of the mentor's role is to give as complete an assessment as possible.

Mentoring need not be limited to those individuals who show specific signs of leadership potential, although certainly this is a good investment in future leaders. In fact, anyone can benefit from a relationship with a mentor, but not everyone will benefit in the same way. The key to making the program work for the newcomer is to find mentors who can adjust their approach to meet the needs of the individual. The ideal mentor will be glad for the opportunity to work with the "raw material" and to help by being responsive to individual needs.

Why Would Staff Want to Mentor?

A successful and enriching mentoring relationship takes time, effort, and lots of energy. Why would health care managers and executives, who already have so many demands on their time and energy, agree to participate in a mentoring program?

First, mentors like to teach, and this is fundamental to a successful program. Members of your management team who enjoy sharing knowledge and ideas, and who enjoy working with others, will be energized by a mentoring relationship. Good mentors recognize the value of testing and exchanging ideas in a risk-free setting. They know that they too will learn by working with new employees who have a new base of knowledge.

The process of mentoring strengthens organizational leadership and continuity. It is not just an accident that many successful fellows and administrative residents end up with their first postfellowship position in the same organization. Mentors realize that mentoring is an opportunity to contribute to young professionals' careers and that, in the process of helping younger administrators succeed, they are helping their own careers as well.

They enjoy working with an energetic new staff member, and they inspire the new member to do excellent work.

In a sense, mentoring is a form of networking; it helps the mentor keep in touch with trends in the environment and expands the newcomer's contacts in the field. Experienced administrators recognize that time spent on developing solid relationships is important throughout one's career. They also realize that even mentors need mentoring, and they build and rely on lifelong contacts with others who are willing to share their expertise. Good mentors who acknowledge this priority are an invaluable resource for incoming employees.

Selecting the Right Staff: Qualities of a Good Mentor

Not every member of your management team who would like to participate in the mentoring program will be cut out for the task. The qualities that contribute to excellence in mentoring are much the same as those contributing to excellence in teaching. Both teachers and mentors understand the virtue of the well-directed question, appreciate persistence in working out logical solutions to problems, and relish the experience of observing individual growth. There is a genuine and overriding interest in the business of "developing" people. Mentors make time to teach. It is not just an assignment, it is an avocation of a high order.

Good mentors teach by example, so they must be emotionally secure individuals who behave in a rational and consistent fashion. The mentor should have high ethical standards and values, supported by the knowledge that value systems established early in a career guide an individual's capacity to lead others to value-based decision making. Mentors serve an important role in upholding organizational standards and setting an example by their own personal and professional integrity.

Developing the Mentoring Relationship

To make the mentoring experience work, the relationship must be developed on a solid basis of mutual trust. The mentor must be willing to take risks, to share thoughts and concepts, and to trust that the information will be kept confidential when appropriate. He or she must be willing to share examples of personal failures as well as successes. The new employee must be able to understand the investment the mentor is making and to trust that the learning process itself will not be judged.

Mentoring requires periods of uninterrupted time and cannot always be dictated by tight schedules. The good mentor is an accessible one. He or she listens carefully and avoids posturing and sermonizing. The mentor should be insightful—able to read between the lines and pick up on the individual's reactions and thoughts.

As the relationship develops, the mentor takes time to reflect on the tasks that have been assigned to the new employee. There should be an attempt to continually increase the newcomer's responsibilities during the formal mentoring relationship. Regular and formal reviews of the new team member's progress, as well as the mentoring relationship itself, are essential. The reviews need to be thorough and candid. Mentoring relationships early in one's career sometimes provide the last significant opportunities for candid reviews, since evaluations tend to become more superficial and political, and therefore less personally valuable, as one's career advances.

Avoiding Pitfalls

What are the major obstacles to the development of a solid mentoring relationship? Perhaps the most inhibiting obstacle is a lack of openness on the part of the mentor. If administrators are unwilling or unable to share enough of themselves, they will not be able to invest adequately in the mentoring process. If the individual being mentored cannot penetrate the mentor's protective shell, it is unlikely that the two will be able to share and confide in one another, and the purpose of the mentoring process will be defeated.

A related obstacle occurs when mentors become preoccupied with their own careers and neglect their responsibilities to the new team member. In some cases, mentors succumb to an overdeveloped personal ego, allowing the relationship to revolve around their own base of knowledge. Obviously, a one-sided relationship is unhealthy because it does not allow the mutual and free exchange of ideas and experiences. A mentor's inability to challenge the individual by asking for opinions is a further indication of a failing relationship, since it probably means that the mentor has little interest in the young professional's ideas.

Another problem occurs if a mentor is not keeping up with current management practices. Mentors need to be on top of events and practices in order to convey knowledge to the new staff member. The mentor's credibility will be impaired if the less-experienced team member recognizes that the mentor's information is not current.

The newcomer's sense of worth and recognition grows in almost direct proportion to the degree of access to the mentor. It is important for those being mentored to be persistent enough to establish regular and consistent interaction with the mentor. On the other hand, a mentor's insensitivity to the newcomer's need to network both within and outside the organization can also create a problem if the mentor monopolizes the new member's time. New employees do not prosper if they are locked up behind the scenes with second-level project work. The mentor should ensure that networking opportunities are available so the new associate enjoys a sufficient degree of visibility and can take advantage of a wide range of experiences working with others in the organization.

Information must flow in both directions, but the mentor must be sensitive to confidentiality issues when sharing information with the newer associate. (The younger associate may not be aware of all of the political ramifications involved.) Others in the organization might welcome the opportunity to hear impressions or comments made by the mentor, but the newcomer's failure to maintain confidences would undermine an otherwise successful relationship. Conversely, a mentor who uses a younger colleague as an organizational spy would obviously ruin the relationship (and reveal the sad state of corporate values).

Mentoring and Teamwork: Issues in Orienting Newcomers

Mentoring provides an excellent opportunity to orient newcomers to the organization's culture, values, and expectations. Careful attention to the orientation of new staff will help the team and the organization as a whole to maintain a unified sense of purpose and direction. Because this relationship is essential to initiating and stimulating creativity among new team members, it is important to look at some of the issues that should be considered in selecting mentors and in anticipating the newcomer's adjustment. Some of the most common issues that arise when new staff are added to an existing team are outlined below. Although they apply most specifically to less experienced and newer team members, they are also relevant to more experienced administrators who enter a new environment.

1. *Problems with time management.* The transition from the academic world to the working world comes as a shock to some young professionals. A newcomer to an organization may experience difficulty in handling multiple projects simultaneously—a reality of the working world. As a mentor, the experienced administrator can help the newcomer by letting the individual know that the time pressure problem is a common condition and by giving suggestions for scheduling each project.

2. *Failure to be specific in assigning tasks.* If the executive is not specific about priorities and the scope of the assignment, the newcomer often will spend too much time and energy completing the

assignment (for example, such as devoting several weeks to a project that only required a quick fix). The newcomer will not know— and should not be expected to know—the level of involvement needed until the leader spells it out in adequate detail.

3. *Underestimation of the impact of operational demands on others.* A new executive might unconsciously make unreasonable demands on others to collect data or information, failing to realize how much effort is required to accomplish the task. This is simply a reflection of the newcomer's desire to succeed and build credibility, but additional work assignments suddenly added to an already heavy work load will not be easily absorbed and will frequently be resented by staff. A mentor can help by informing the new team member of work flow patterns and demands on staff time, and by providing suggestions for how to time special requests of staff.

4. *Lack of awareness of organizational relationships.* Newcomers sometimes overlook the importance of assessing the organizational culture before charging into unknown waters. In some ways, organizational charts are like road maps. Both identify major routes, but unlike organizational charts road maps also show alternate routes to destinations. Since organizational charts only show official relationships, they sometimes mislead newcomers. Actual relationships between executives are much more important than how the relationship looks on paper. Newcomers need to spend time learning about these relationships, and leaders have a responsibility to spend enough time with them to provide this essential orientation.

5. *Inappropriate expectation levels.* Another common problem is that the new team member often underestimates the amount of time it takes to establish personal credibility. Previous experience and academic credentials do not carry much weight with new colleagues. The newcomer must earn the respect of the rest of the team. In addition, the authority and power that the newcomer has inherited by virtue of his or her new position in the organization should be applied with sensitivity, wisdom, and judgment. Applying authority thoughtfully will enhance the individual's credibility and ability to meet other people's expectations. A good mentor will help the new team member to understand the expectations of the rest of the team.

6. *Inadequate implementation of ideas.* One very important asset that newcomers bring to the organization is their unique knowledge and experience. Sometimes newcomers transfer this knowledge (about

new technology, for example) without being conscious of the fact that their method of offering information threatens existing staff members. New tools learned in the classroom or in other institutions need to be used thoughtfully. On the other hand, it is unfortunate that, after a year or two, many new executives forget or ignore their previously acquired skills. The older team members' inertia and the newcomer's desire to be accepted can combine to inhibit the newcomer's ability to contribute to the change process. The mentor who values new insight but understands the rest of the staff's point of view can encourage positive, nonthreatening outlets for the newcomer's creative energy and ideas, and can give directions for the appropriate timing for introducing new information.

7. *Isolation.* Another frustration faced by newcomers is that they fail to recognize that chief executive officers, dealing with many different issues, may not always be easily accessible for counseling, support, and direction. This creates a sense of isolation. The mentoring relationship helps to alleviate this problem, in part by urging the new member to merge successfully into team processes by keeping in close contact with many others in the organization.

8. *Failure to network.* As projects and activities accelerate, some new staff members have a tendency to retreat to focus on specific projects and to get work done. This is unfortunate. It is important that individuals circulate freely within the new organization and that they develop contacts with peers in other organizations. All of these contacts should be maintained and strengthened continually. Outside exposure is vital because it provides important environmental surveillance input that allows ideas developed elsewhere to be applied internally. A good mentor will keep an eye on the newcomer and try to ensure that specific project demands do not deter the individual from seeking information and input from outside the organization.

9. *Retention of self-centered ideas.* Sometimes new members of the team arrive thinking that the organization should change its ways to accommodate them and that such change should occur easily and naturally. Obviously, change does not work this way. Personal sacrifice is necessary in lasting relationships, and early adjustment to the organizational climate will help the newcomer to develop trusting relationships with team members. Once trust has been established, innovation will occur more rapidly through the group process, and new ideas will be more readily accepted. The mentor can help with this adjustment by talking with the newcomer about the dynamics

and orientation of the team, and by giving advice on how to express suggestions for change.

The Maturing Mentoring Relationship

Being a mentor means more than just having individuals seek you out for information. Ideally, mentoring is an effort to develop a very close relationship with another individual; it involves sharing thoughts and concerns, and approaches to decision making. At times, the closeness can create a sense of mutual dependency. Seasoned mentors understand this and, as the new associate matures, will seek ways to carefully disengage a bit—to stand back from the process and allow the less experienced colleague to develop independently.

However, the solid mentoring relationship need not be severed altogether. In fact, some mentoring relationships are maintained over a period of years or throughout one's career. But care should be taken by both parties to avoid excessive dependency. Care should also be taken to ensure that the mentoring relationship does not irritate others in the organization. The health care leader should monitor the impact that the relationship has on others in the organization, guarding against any perception of undue favoritism, which could serve to undermine the development of a total team effort.

Conclusion

The mentoring process is complex, but the relationship provides positive, professional growth for both parties. The best mentoring situation is one that encourages introspection, self-awareness, and a considerable amount of hard work. When mentoring works well, it is the result of a considerable investment of energy by both parties.

Note

1. M. Zey, *The Mentor Connection* (New Brunswick, NJ: Transaction Publications, 1990).

6

MAINTAINING MORALE: CONFRONTATION, EVALUATION, AND COMPENSATION

Case in Point

John Coatsworth was an excellent assistant administrator at Davenport General Medical Center, a 600-bed tertiary care unit. His supervisors liked working with him. In every respect except one, John excelled. His only weakness was that he found it very difficult to do written annual evaluations of those he supervised. As a result, when it came time to set new compensation levels, his team members were at a disadvantage because the records did not justify the amount of the increases he recommended.

Davenport's associate administrator, Nancy Updyke, decided to lay it on the line and insist that John meet organizational requirements regarding the evaluation process. She called a meeting with John to confront him on the matter, and the outcome was very interesting.

John's defense of his behavior was based on two principles. The first was that he resisted highly structured annual evaluations because he felt that the managers he supervised needed and deserved reinforcement and encouragement year-round. The formal end-of-the-year review process gave an artificial flavor to what he felt should be an ongoing evaluation process. His second argument was equally compelling. Annual evaluations tended to have a negative tone. One was expected to praise the staff member for good behavior but then to find things that needed to be improved. As a result, the annual reviews tended to end on a slightly sour note.

John also pointed out that he did not believe that detailed documentation of performance on an annual basis was very worthwhile, particularly since his administrative colleagues were creating evaluation reports that served to artificially inflate the worth of their staff members. Administrators were, in effect, distorting evaluations to enhance the perceived value of their own team members. This did little to encourage other staff members to contribute their best work, or to reward them fairly and sincerely for their efforts.

Following their meeting, Nancy thought about this at length and arrived at some interesting conclusions. First, John was right. The system was being manipulated. Second, evaluations should be ongoing and not conducted at artificially set schedules. Third, the format of the required evaluation focused on detailed performance criteria, not necessarily on those items that could make a difference in overall performance. (For example, the manager's ability to perform technical evaluations of his or her staff members was given the same weight as the manager's demonstration of leadership in seeking out solutions to problems.)

As a result of Nancy's assessment (and John's honesty), the evaluation process was redesigned to focus on continuous feedback, and the criteria were simplified to identify those characteristics that really could make a difference. John, in response, agreed to conform to the need for documenting performance evaluations, and committed himself to helping to structure a process to ensure resolution of internal equity and compensation issues.

No matter how well a team works together, there will always be concerns and issues related to individual performance that the leader must address. Particularly stressful conditions are likely to draw even greater attention to these matters, and the health care system is certainly full of stressful conditions. The way in which the leader chooses to address some of the more sensitive and personal issues involved in directing staff members will have a significant effect on the morale and performance of the team as a whole, as well as on the individual members.

Confrontation

Confrontation in management is an attempt to force sensitive or destructive issues out into the open so individuals can begin the healing process necessary to put the issues behind them. Because the result of confrontation is not usually predictable, leaders should be judicious in their use of confrontation as a management tool. Leaders should always size up all the options for addressing a particular problem or situation before deciding to confront.

Most people—including most leaders—shy away from interpersonal conflict. But avoiding confrontation in an organizational setting encourages guerrilla warfare. Much energy is wasted by circumventing conflicts that, if they were confronted directly, might result in solutions that would free up the parties involved and allow them to engage in more productive behavior. It is the leader's responsibility to maximize effectiveness within the organization, and sometimes this means making sure that confrontation occurs.

Complicated organizations such as health care institutions, which are staffed by a wide variety of professional, technical, and support staff, have the potential for a considerable amount of role conflict. Health care executives who work constantly to pull these diverse and potentially competing elements together may fear that confronting conflict will only serve to create additional controversy, thus further dividing their staff. In addition, because the pace of the health care institution is so hectic, health care executives are usually trying to conserve and ration staff energy (both physical and psychic). Those who think that confrontation requires more energy than simply avoiding the conflict will often opt for the latter approach.

Who and When to Confront

Sometimes the leader is not the best person to confront an issue. Administrators who do not have enough technical or scientific expertise to address professional conflicts between technical or scientific staff should probably not use confrontation as a management technique in those situations. Professionals might resent an executive's intrusion in an area where he or she lacks the background needed to assess the situation, and they might be more capable of resolving the problem or disagreement without intervention.

For example, physicians often are willing to debate differences of opinion with each other without making an emotional investment in the process. In most cases, they are challenging each other to determine the appropriate treatment approach or other course of action to take on behalf of a patient. They all know that the ultimate resolution of the issue will be up to the physician in charge of the patient's care. However, their ability to debate the issue with each other generates less heat and fire than there would be if the responsible physician were approached by an executive without a clinical orientation.

Confrontations with board members are delicate matters for health care leaders. Not only do board members bring different skills, personalities, interests, and talents to the playing field, they are also responsible for the recruiting, nourishing, and, if necessary, the firing of the CEO. There are occasions when executives are sorely tested by the unevenness of this playing field. For example, how should the CEO respond to a conflict of interest in a member of the board? It takes a great deal of courage for the CEO to remember that confronting may incur the wrath of the board member but that overlooking the conflict of interest will mean losing the game entirely.

In some situations, direct confrontation may not be the best solution. The CEO might maintain more credibility by trying to orchestrate an indirect intervention. One way of anticipating and monitoring conflicts of interest is the routine practice of requiring that a conflict-of-interest questionnaire be filed annually by all board members and management with a board committee, to identify any possible relationships that might put the individual and the organization in either financial or ethical conflict. By anticipating the conflict in advance and using peer pressure to resolve issues, the CEO is able to establish norms for board-directed policies and at the same time to avoid unnecessary confrontation with the board. When this type of prevention is not possible, however, the CEO's value system will probably be put to the test.

Level of risk. When determining whether or not to confront a particular managerial issue, leaders should consider the level of risk inherent in the confrontation. If the confrontation addresses the personality or ego of an individual, it will carry personal implications that do not come into play when addressing a clearly defined organizational problem. Poor managerial performance obviously needs to be confronted, but the wise executive will gather the facts and determine the level of confrontation needed based on whether the issues are internal and within the individual's control (e.g., style of management) or external and beyond the individual's control (e.g., an adverse ruling by a state agency on a certificate-of-need request for a new lung transplant program). When the parties involved in a conflict are not at an equal level in the organization's hierarchy, the lower-ranking staff member will obviously feel most at risk in a confrontation with the higher-ranking member. It is important that the executive anticipate the effect of these differences ahead of time.

Timing. The executive also has to consider timing. When is the correct time to confront a situation? The right time to confront is more apparent when less risky problem-solving practices have been tried without success, or when the problem worsens and is clearly interfering with the organization's operations. When aberrant behavior undermines the value system or the ethics of the organization, rapid intercession is essential.

Timing may also depend on the environmental circumstances affecting the organization. Confrontation usually is more urgent if the organization is facing difficult times (financial or otherwise) and decisions have to be made quickly. But the health care executive who employs confrontation as an active tool needs to develop an ability to see beyond the immediate crisis in order to anticipate the outcome. Executives must approach confrontation with their own emotions in check if they want to be in the best position to control the process and not be trapped into responding inappropriately to personal attacks. This also means being willing to take the risks associated with an adverse outcome to the process.

Using Appropriate Channels

Occasionally a member of the staff will exercise a management style designed to deflect other staff members. Signals are sent out that others should stay clear of that individual's agenda or suffer the consequences, which may be rudeness, harsh statements, or other antisocial behavior. This style of intimidation is subtle but destructive, and the leader who observes such practices should not let them go unconfronted. Remember, however, that senior executives are not always privy to these behavioral patterns, even if the behaviors are obvious to others. Some excellent leaders may be accused by staff of avoiding conflict when in fact they are either unaware of the problem or unaware that it is so severe. Leaders must have multiple channels of input. They must work hard to observe, to "manage by walking around," and to keep in touch by developing formal and informal methods of obtaining input on managerial behavior.

If the facts suggest that a problem needs to be resolved, the thoughtful leader should look for opportunities to confront the issue through the appropriate channels. If the misbehaving member of the team is two levels down in the organization, the leader should deal directly with the individual's direct supervisor. The executive should first determine whether or not the individual is indeed out of line, and then why the individual's supervisor has not taken corrective action.

Many individuals who create personal or organizational problems are highly competent on the job and simply need some individual counseling. Others, however, need to be warned that although they are competent, their behavior cannot be tolerated, and unless the behavior improves they will have to be terminated. This type of confrontation should be direct and straightforward. Leaders who are obtuse and indirect often fail to convey the seriousness of the confrontation, yet these situations must be solved before the team is eroded. It is the leader's responsibility to intervene to remove obstacles that are inhibiting the team's ability to get its job done. And the leader's supporters (secretaries, managers, supervisors, and others), who are usually well aware of performance problems, will be watching carefully to see if the executive is willing to handle such behavior.

Suggestions Regarding the Confrontation Process

There are a few key steps in preparing for confrontation. First, be sure that the problem has been diagnosed accurately and has been examined from various viewpoints. For example, has an individual's behavior pattern changed recently because of some particular organizational or personal stress, or is it a management style or personality problem? (If it is a style or personality problem, it will be harder to resolve.) When assessing the problem, be careful not to assume that individuals who are behaving poorly are aware that they are doing so. Poor behavior may be related to a practice style that was acceptable when the individual was working in another organization and setting.

Second, begin to bring the issue out in the open with those closest to the problem and listen carefully for reasons why the individual's behavior is being tolerated. This sets the stage for problem resolution. Then determine the conditions required for acceptable performance. If those directly responsible for resolving a problem (for example, a chief of staff who should be dealing with a medical staff problem) are unwilling or uncomfortable with the confrontation, collaborate to develop a joint program leading to confrontation.

Once confrontation has occurred, be sure to establish schedules for reviewing progress to measure changes in behavior. If you (or the individual's supervisor) indicate to the individual that progress will be reviewed in 30 or 60 days, make sure you do not miss the deadline. Once the confrontation process begins, it must be followed through to an ultimate conclusion, and this requires honest and timely feedback.

When performance has improved (and it usually does), be sure to take the heat off the individual by making it clear that the problem has been resolved. It is unfair to leave a sanctioned action (such as possible loss of position) hanging over an individual's head indefinitely. If the problem has not been resolved within the time limit, then take the action that was planned, but never leave the individual wondering whether or not there has been any change in your perception of his or her performance.

Evaluation

Health care leaders must pay very close attention to the processes of evaluating and rewarding colleagues and staff, as well as ensuring that those processes are functioning elsewhere in the organization. Although the suggestions made in this section will focus specifically on evaluating and rewarding the performance of the management group, most of the practices outlined can also be applied at other levels in the organization.

The key to effective evaluation practices is keeping accurate and updated position descriptions. These descriptions provide points of reference against which an individual's performance can be measured fairly and objectively. In a volatile environment jobs change continually. Staff should be asked to update their position descriptions regularly, and their descriptions should be discussed with them and then officially accepted. Without up-to-date job descriptions as a basis for comparison, leaders and managers will have to redefine evaluation criteria at every performance review.

Of course, the job of keeping position descriptions current does not rest only with the CEO or supervisor. The associate administrator in a skilled nursing facility who wants to be recognized for taking on new community responsibilities should make sure that those new responsibilities are recorded. Most health care organizations have their own formal guidelines for listing, evaluating, and updating performance objectives.

Evaluation Criteria for Managers

At higher levels in the organization it may be more difficult to provide precise, objective criteria for purposes of evaluation. The broad area of responsibility assigned to upper management usually carries broad expectations, and so evaluation criteria are also difficult to pin down. How does one evaluate, for example, the CEO's ability to keep the organization viable and progressive rather than stagnating? In spite of what sometimes seem like intangible responsibilities, it is important to penetrate generalities and work to define specific, objective criteria. Therefore, when evaluating members of the management team, the leader should supplement any formal organizational criteria that do exist with criteria that will reflect performance on strategic leadership and management issues. The criteria should reflect issues such as those listed below:

- Does the manager personally confront problems in a timely fashion and, in the process, exercise good judgment? (Or does the executive avoid personal involvement and risk by inappropriately relying on subordinates to confront others?)

- What about the executive's competence in processing complex issues? Does the manager possess the intellectual capacity to wrestle with an entire strategy? (Or does the executive only look at the next step in the process?)

- How is the executive perceived by his or her peers in terms of leadership? Does the manager rank well among other executives with the same level of experience? Is the executive respected and valued as a person of high integrity? (Or does the executive "just get by"?)

- Is the executive truly a team leader? Are strong members of the team successfully recruited and retained? Is there team continuity, mutual respect, and interdependence? (Or does the executive try to be surrounded by team members who will agree with the leader without providing direct and honest input in decision making?)

- What about the team member's level of self-awareness? Is the executive able to see the big picture? (Or does the executive consistently translate events only as they seem personally relevant—which might suggest a problem of an oversized ego?)

- Is the executive able to explain complex affairs to boards, management, medical staff, and employees? Are written and verbal skills average, above average, or superior? (Or is the executive dependent on colleagues to pull together the presentations and carry the weight of the dialogue?)

- How does the executive's overall track record look? Has performance been consistent? (Or is there a lack of consistent performance in matters of judgment?)

- Is the manager truly keeping up with new professional developments through active participation in continuing education and involvement in professional societies? Does the executive network well externally? (Or does the executive rely on past practices as the only way to solve a problem, or follow a practice of professional isolation?)

- How effective is the executive as a teacher or mentor? Does the team member display enthusiasm in interchanges with colleagues, managers, students, and others? (Or does the executive communicate that teaching and mentoring are an extra burden—a task to be assigned to others?)

- Does the executive use a single standard for evaluating and rewarding others in the organization in order to ensure equity, and does the team member evaluate employees objectively according to actual performance? (Or does the executive follow a double standard and display signs of favoritism in making such decisions?)

- What about the executive's personal ethics and values? Is there understanding and ongoing demonstration of ethical behavior? Does the executive operate with respect for and belief in the rights and welfare of others, regardless of their position in the organization? Is there honesty in relationships with colleagues?

- Are the executive's performance and behavior perceived as complementary to the mission of the organization? Is the individual loyal? Is the executive known for objectivity, or are biases displayed to others?

The contemporary health care leader needs to spend time contemplating all of these questions (and others as well) when designing a philosophy of leadership that encourages a thorough and exacting process of evaluation of the executives (including the leader) in the organization.

Timing, Procedures, and Processes

Members of the management team should be formally evaluated at least once each year. However, concurrent and continuous evaluations should supplement annual reviews. To put it simply: pluses and minuses should not be tallied for a whole year before they are ever discussed. There should be an open dialogue regarding performance, and that will require constant monitoring and ongoing communication.

One technique that will assist in the evaluation process is to ask individuals to complete a self-assessment. A self-assessment should be based on criteria selected jointly with the individual's supervisor. Each party should complete the evaluation, and the two should then meet to compare and discuss ratings and rankings. This process is more interactive, allowing both individuals an opportunity to express their perceptions, rather than simply having the supervisor complete the written evaluation, schedule a meeting, and talk through the evaluation.

Another process that can be both useful and revealing, although it might be perceived as more threatening, is to have managers select individuals to complete an anonymous evaluation of their performance. The goal is to obtain honest input on performance, so managers must be willing to take the risk of learning about their own performance problems! Obviously, this process can only be used successfully in an organization with a high level of trust among its staff.

Regardless of the approach to the actual evaluation, the criteria used to evaluate staff members should always be shared with them in advance, and copies of results of interviews and the annual performance evaluations should be provided to the individual being interviewed. Verbal and written feedback are both critical to the process.

Evaluating the CEO: The Role of the Governing Board

Unfortunately, these days health services executives often find the security of their own positions to be tenuous. Part of the problem lies in the inability of some governing boards to implement effective evaluation processes for the CEO. Health care executives need to work to educate and orient their governing boards regarding the importance of this responsibility. Some executives may be uncomfortable with helping to orchestrate the evaluation process, and this is understandable. But it is also shortsighted. Without established evaluation criteria and processes, the executive is subject to the whims of board members. Making sure that the processes are in place ultimately may turn out to be a step toward self-preservation.

Compensation

Directing the internal affairs of a health services organization is a trying and challenging assignment, and outstanding performance needs to be rewarded through recognition and adequate compensation. Five or ten years ago, the level of compensation for health care executives was significantly lower than for executives in other industries. Fortunately, industries—including health care—have learned that it is important to make the financial investment needed to recruit and retain the best minds, particularly in troubled times.

Today compensation of health care executives is rising more rapidly than some anticipated, in spite of the financial turmoil being experienced in the field. In addition to increasing salaries, more and more health care organizations are developing incentive (bonus) programs, which help to recognize the efforts of individuals on their management teams. These programs are designed to reward individuals and teams for achieving predetermined financial and service goals. They are very difficult to implement in health care because so much of the end result depends on team effort rather than individual performance. The incentive systems that appear to work the best are those that reward group effort and serve to build collaborative efforts, as contrasted with those designed to reward solo performers.

Internal Equity

Leaders also need to pay close attention to compensation equity at the other levels in the organization. Everybody is interested in their fair share, no matter what their salary grade. Particularly in multiunit organizations, where units are closely interrelated (e.g., hospitals and group practices), senior executives have a very special role in monitoring the compensation systems in subsidiary organizations to ensure that rankings and values are dispensed equitably. Marketplace compensation surveys are useful, but since job descriptions usually vary substantially, judgment is needed to determine appropriate compensation levels for similar positions. Market surveys will probably not exactly match the organization's positions, but over time the leader will develop a feeling for what is fair and come up with figures that seem right. This is not a very scientific process so the leader will need to balance organizational guidelines for internal equity, standards in the marketplace, and instinct for what is fair.

Compensation must be based on performance, and failure to reward appropriately will lead to a breakdown of morale and dissension within the team. While salary information should be considered confidential, individuals within organizations have an incredible ability to find out about inequities. The organizational grapevine is particularly active when it comes to compensation. The wise leader recognizes this inclination and takes careful steps to ensure equity and fairness.

Contracts for Administrators

Another way for leaders to recognize the efforts of excellent managers is to negotiate protection through the use of employment contracts. Ten or fifteen years ago it was considered undignified to require an employment contract; a simple handshake as a sign of good faith was considered enough. Even today, organizations that espouse strong values and have an appreciation for the need to protect decision makers in the organization may not need to rely on contracts with employees. However, as leaders in the health care field have encountered more and more conditions in which difficult (and sometimes risky) decisions have had to be made, the benefit of contracts has become more apparent.

A contract protects both the organization and the individual executive. For the organization, the contract ensures that the terms of employment have been spelled out and that the conditions for separation are known. By issuing a contract, the organization is giving the executive license to make tough decisions, license that will be needed in order to reach organizational objectives. However, if the organization wants out of the contract for some reason, all parties will know the cost of that decision. By accepting a contract, the executive is acknowledging that he or she understands the parameters of the arrangement as well as the expectations that come along with it. The executive who is backed up and protected by a contract might be more willing to take the necessary risks on behalf of the organization without running scared. Leadership strategies in the years ahead will require additional risk taking, and executives must be protected so they will be willing to do what it takes to move the organization forward.

Conclusion

The way in which a leader addresses personnel issues—confrontation, evaluation, compensation—has a tremendous impact on individual and team morale within the organization. Promoting a positive team spirit does not necessarily mean giving team members everything they want. It does mean, however, that the leader is willing to confront problems that affect the staff so the staff will have confidence that their concerns will be understood and that they will be treated fairly and consistently. Team members at every level must be assured that they serve a vital role in the organization if they are to feel that they are important contributors to the team. The leader who can handle sensitive personnel issues straightforwardly will contribute much to the growth of productive teams.

7

A TEAM APPROACH TO
STRATEGIC PLANNING

Case in Point

Like many other organizations, Virginia Mason Medical Center had always looked at strategic planning as an upper management activity. Leaders at the top of the organization would meet to develop a plan and move it along through the usual approval process. As the health care environment began to change, however, competition and other financial pressures were such that the strategic plan could no longer be considered a concern that applied only to the organization's senior executives. Staff at every level in the organization would be affected by the strategic plan, and it no longer made sense for a few to decide the destiny of the organization without serious input from the stakeholders. We needed a totally new approach to planning that would include as many board members, medical staff members, and employees as possible.

Although some staff felt strongly that it would be most efficient for top medical, managment, and board leaders to simply go off on a retreat and come back with a plan, we decided that our goal should be organization-wide involvement. So in 1989 we began a six-month planning process that was internally facilitated, well staffed, and outcome oriented, setting the stage for the organization's next leap forward. The exercise not only produced a new plan but also energized the organization and assisted in furthering organizational integration and a sense of renewal. This process of extended involvement has become a part of the organization's culture and is still used every time the strategic plan is updated.

Health care executives are often frustrated with strategic planning. It is a complicated process that consumes a considerable amount of organizational energy and that has to be repeated if it is to remain current and useful. The unique relationships between the medical staff, the board, and management make the strategic planning process in health care quite complicated, and those who lead the planning exercise do not necessarily have the authority to direct the outcome, as would be more typical in the business and commercial environment. This chapter centers on a way to approach strategic planning that reaps the rewards of team building by involving the entire team in investing in and directing the organization.

Despite our frustration with the process, strategic planning is absolutely essential for organizational survival, and the health care executive who wants to lead an organization into the twenty-first century must be able to work with a management team that can contend with this endeavor. One of the benefits of working with a mature team is being able to rely on it for input into future directions. Strategic planning is the means by which an organization develops a vision of what it would like to be and then plots the means to get there. The analysis, evaluation, speculation, and vision required to complete the process determine the nature and the direction that the organization should take.

Strategic Planning in the Health Care Environment

In the 1960s, strategic planning in health care was facilities oriented. Organizations developed strategies around the extension, expansion, or replacement of existing hospital structures. The planning basically centered on projecting historical data (for example, patient admissions) into the future to forecast the organizational capacity required to accommodate increased volume. This was an appropriate planning posture in the 1960s because the future was reasonably predictable.

In the 1970s, the process changed. Planning was still facilities oriented, but it became programmatic in nature. Organizations' strategic plans contained more substantive material regarding the function housed in each organizational facility. Improved forecasting techniques led to an increase in the number of alternatives included in strategic plans, which allowed greater flexibility for adopting new technologies.

Planning in the 1970s was still based on assumptions of continuous growth and was driven by the level of planning processes required through federal and state regulations. The certificate of need required by hospitals to build new facilities or add new services was an example of such a regulation. Although these regulations forced organizations to look further into the future, they also had the undesirable effect of accelerating construction and facility development by increasing competition for future opportunities.

In the 1980s, the environment began to change rapidly as market and competitive forces surfaced with a vengeance. Incentives also changed. Hospital executives began to refine and respond to new reimbursement systems (diagnosis-related groups) that rewarded organizations that could move patients out of the hospital rapidly. Managed health care systems matured and hospitals or health systems lost large groups of patients as employers cut new contracts with other systems for caring for those patients. Capital resources became more limited, which made decision making regarding new technology much more difficult than in the past. As the future became less predictable, it was essential for organizations to further increase their flexibility to adapt to these changes. Leaders began to focus more on providing vision and direction for the organization, allowing room for maneuvering and for mid-course adjustments.

Strategic planning in the 1990s needs to focus on even more general goals for the organization. Too much locking in on details can lead organizations to short-term strategies that might hamper their flexibility and ability to respond to significant environmental changes. Robert Hayes explains this approach by noting, "When you are lost on the highway, a road map is very useful; but when you are lost in the swamp, whose topography is constantly changing, a road map is of little help. A simple compass—which indicates the general direction to be taken, and allows you to use your own ingenuity in overcoming various obstacles—is much more valuable."[1]

The problem most of us have with strategic planning is that we cannot guarantee that our forecast for the future is accurate. Fortunately, the use of multiple scenarios (the description of possible future events in terms of best and worst case scenarios) for forecasting a future course of events is becoming more common in health services planning. This discipline, based on careful use of data and supplemented by intuitive guesses or forecasts about given points in the future, has made the process somewhat more scientific. However, even at its best, strategic planning is still a best guess among options.

Still, we have little choice but to use strategic planning to chart our course in a changing environment. Organizations that think of strategic planning as a way of dealing with change are able to adapt. For example, the Perkins School for the Blind in Watertown, Massachusetts, which was opened in the 1800s, had a clear-cut charter to educate blind school-age boys of normal intelligence.[2] By 1960, however, there were fewer and fewer children with the single handicap of blindness. The majority of blind people were middle-aged or older, and many children who were blind also had other handicaps. To adapt to these changing circumstances, the Perkins

School revamped its charter to include children of both sexes with multiple handicaps. The organization took a realistic look at current and predictable conditions and determined how they would have to adapt in order to survive. For many of us in health care, planning in the next decade will have an equally serious focus.

The Strategic Planning Process

Getting Ready

The leader needs to accomplish six tasks before the planning process itself begins. During the planning process, the CEO should monitor and revise the elements involved in these six specific tasks.

The first responsibility is to assemble the planning team and establish its responsibilities. This involves much more than simply gathering a group and telling them to go to it. An agenda of events needs to be carefully prepared. The planning process must be subdivided into digestible segments and leaders who possess facilitating skills should be identified for work on each segment. Expectations must be identified in advance. Advance notice of the process and its importance must be carefully communicated throughout the organization. The way in which key players in the organization get involved in the process of planning will be crucial to the acceptance of the plan and its subsequent implementation. The team should include physicians, governing board members, senior executives, managers, and others, depending on their skills and capabilities. However, the planning structure cannot be unwieldy and the total process must be conducted without prejudging the outcome.

In large health care organizations, the CEO might want to develop several different committees: a steering committee of approximately eight or nine members, subcommittees to work on specific issues, and a larger planning review committee to serve in the role of overseer. In smaller health units, structures have to be sized accordingly, but the principle of maximizing the number of staff members involved is still a valid concept, in spite of the extra energy that it requires to ensure meaningful involvement from many.

The second task is to develop the time lines for the process. Obviously the first round of developing a brand new strategic plan will take more time than will the annual task of updating the plans. It is best to have tight time lines established at the front end of the process, even if they are extended later. A master calendar should be marked with target dates and functions, and the time lines should be monitored regularly.

The third task, which should be designed even in advance of the main planning effort, is for the CEO to think through the ratification process of the plan. How will the plan be presented for board approval? What are the steps necessary to involve members of the medical staff, not only ensuring their input but ensuring ratification of the end result? What is the best way to obtain input and review from special groups (i.e., professional nurses, pharmacists, and others)?

The fourth task is to determine the sequencing of the planning process. Again, the CEO's role is not to dictate sequencing issues but to make sure that those who are most capable of establishing the sequence are involved in the process. Sequencing is making decisions about which parts of the planning process to undertake at which time. For example, organizations often determine their missions as one of the very first steps in strategic planning. On the other hand, some choose to delay the definition of their mission (which is usually a revision of an existing mission statement) until some of the environmental assessment activities have been completed. Rapid changes in the health care environment justify the decision to shift the sequence of steps. Failing to wait until the environment is sized up before developing the mission statement might result in a mission that would drive the strategic plan in a direction that would be undermined by prohibitive external factors.

The fifth step is to determine how the results of the strategic planning process will be disseminated. The plan will contain a certain amount of proprietary information, which in today's competitive arena may need to be handled on a confidential basis. Yet the point of involving members of the employee and professional staffs, as well as members of the governing board, is that wider dissemination and feedback are essential to building momentum for implementation of the plan. The senior executive and management team need to clearly understand the risks of disseminating too much information, as well as the risks of failing to do so. (As a general rule, the dissemination of more information, rather than less, is better.)

Finally, the sixth task is to establish how the plan will be evaluated once it is implemented. What criteria should be used to determine whether or not the plan is meeting the organization's needs, and further, at what intervals should the plan be updated?

Collaborating with Professional Planners

Setting up integrated planning teams, which include professionals with both planning and executive skills, makes a lot more sense than delegating the development of a strategic plan to a planning group. Planners should be in the mainstream of the operation; otherwise the outcome of the planning might not hold up when actually put to the test. Professional planners and operations executives tend to approach things very differently. When their efforts are not synchronized and integrated, they frequently come into conflict. Some of the resulting attitudes and experiences are noted in Exhibit 7.1.

Strategic Planning Events

Strategic planning begins with a thorough environmental assessment, which includes an inventory of the external environment, the competition, and health service trends. It is followed by the definition or refinement of the organization's mission statement. This requires consideration of how the mission statement will be used, who it is being written for (i.e., the external patient group or the internal employee force), and how long it should be. (An example of a mission statement is included in Chapter 2.)

Based on the external assessment of the mission, the market and service mix are analyzed. This analysis is basically an internal environmental assessment incorporating careful evaluation of medical, surgical, and obstetrical services, and their trend lines and forecasts for the future based on staff availability and needs. New health services programs are examined, and the mix between inpatient and ambulatory services is studied.

This is the most time-consuming and complicated part of the strategic planning process. The immediate organization and implementation of this stage might take three to four months to complete, but the implementation of an action plan could take several years. The process involves building blocks of information, integrating the information into specific digestible projects, and moving the program forward.

Special subgroups may be assigned to study specific topics that will be incorporated into the strategic plan. Groups might be charged either with the study of practice patterns to determine responsiveness to reimbursement systems, or with technology assessment to predict types of technology that will need to be replaced and new technology that should be acquired in the years ahead. The process might even include the development of a method for determining how technology is assessed. There may be special studies of service aspects of the organization as well as studies of the effectiveness of internal communication systems (i.e., whether the medical staff is being kept involved and informed).

A major complaint with strategic planning in these days of diminishing resources is with the difficulty of building financial scenarios. The strategic planning process addresses a number of questions related to the organization's financial status and interests for the future. Do we have a five-year capital acquisition plan? How much debt can we tolerate? What financial ratios should be established as targets?

The organization's governance and organizational structures must also be addressed. Is the board properly constituted and of the right size for

Exhibit 7.1 Why Professional Planners and Operations Executives Need Integrated Strategic Planning: Common Issues and Contrasting Concerns

Planners' Concerns	Issue	Operations Executives' Concerns
"I plan but no one listens, or I am the last to hear of new, budding programs. They simply don't seem to want to include me in the process."	COMMUNICATION	"Planners are out of touch with reality. Why don't they network better and learn what's really coming down?"
"We always seem to conduct our planning without having adequate resources. Doesn't management understand the amount of time it takes to produce what they ask for?"	TIME PRESSURES	"We have to operate with tight time constraints, and planners always look for solutions with a 100 percent guarantee. We don't have time for that luxury. We need to focus on workable options."
"Administrators are so involved in day-to-day operations that they base their priorities on solving yesterday's problems. They don't look far enough into the future."	PRIORITIES	"We see too much reliance on data. Sometimes you have to make decisions based on instincts."
"Even when I develop a good plan and turn it over to operations, it doesn't seem to get implemented. Sometimes it even gets sabotaged."	AUTHORITY	"Why do planners often think that plans can be implemented so easily? We have to find the resources, motivate the staff, and set the stage before implementation begins and too frequently we are surprised with unexpected recommendations."

Continued

Exhibit 7.1   Continued

Planners' Concerns	Issue	Operations Executives' Concerns
"Priorities constantly shift around here so I really don't know the agenda. How can I plan if no one tells me what they see from the top of the tower?"	DIRECTION	"Planners really don't understand how the place works. We can't drop everything to implement a new project or plan. Planning has to fit into the big picture, and its my responsibility to set priorities, not theirs."
"Our planning processes are convoluted. Someone has an idea, someone else changes the direction, and by the time a decision is reached, the essence of the idea has been lost. Our bureaucracy wraps up good ideas and buries them."	DECISION MAKING	"Timing is an essential ingredient. Some of our best strategies have to remain under wraps until we have the support rallied to make it work. Planners sometimes become impatient because they don't understand what it takes to move strategic issues through complex decision-making processes."

maximum effectiveness and efficiency? Are management processes integrated and well directed? Are governance and organizational evaluation processes in place and working? Are the respective roles of governance and management clearly delineated? Are personnel shortages and other issues being addressed?

Obviously, the success of the strategic planning process depends a lot on how well the management team sets up and supports the exercise from beginning to end. It is important that the roles of the team members be clarified. Everyone should know who is in control of the process and how much involvement the CEO will have (as well as how much detail the CEO will expect in reporting).

The staff resources needed to conduct a thorough process must be identified early so that there are no surprises. Even the frequency of update meetings, where key players exchange information on progress, needs to be spelled out. The entire process works best when all members of the management team are focused and truly functioning as a team.

The Role of the Chief Executive Officer

Because organizations cannot predict the future with great safety, CEOs have a difficult role in leading the strategic planning process. The role of the CEO is to assemble the planning team, establish the ground rules and time table, and oversee the process itself. The CEO monitors the process sufficiently to ensure that positive results occur, that the plan receives full review and approval throughout the organization, and that it is ultimately implemented.

One of the mistakes made by many senior executives is that they believe that they must control, rather than simply coordinate and monitor, the planning process. Too frequently executives will closet themselves with four or five key members of the management team and "develop" a strategic plan, which is then unveiled with great ceremony. Imposing a plan designed by the executive staff alone deprives the organization of the kind of synergy and focus that characterizes organizations in which planning is an open process and many groups in the organization have solid and meaningful input. Organizations that take shortcuts in strategic planning (by limiting involvement) should not be surprised if the plan is not wholeheartedly accepted by those who must implement it at different levels in the organization.

Senior executives play a vital role by nudging the organization toward the vision on the horizon. They are in an invaluable position to identify external environmental conditions and broad-based internal issues that need to be addressed in the planning process. The following examples from outside the health care arena may help to illuminate the goal that leaders should have in facilitating the process:

About every ten years, the president of a major home building corporation in Japan issues a memorandum informing all employees and staff members that he is dead. He then lays low and expects the company to respond by reassessing assignments of key people or by challenging old programs and coming up with new ideas. If one of his executives comes to him and tells him that a subsidiary is doing well under the present program, he will say: "That's the way it used to be before the president died. Can't you find a better way to do it?"

The turnaround of the Ford Motor Company several years ago may have had something to do with executives who grasped the fact that the worker on the assembly line probably knew what was wrong with the old Ford. It was reported that the senior executive could regularly be seen riding one of the cars down the assembly line as it was being assembled, asking employees on the spot for their thoughts on how the job could be done more effectively.

The secret to strategic planning, if there is one, is to "work the crowd." People want to be part of a winning team. They must understand where the organization is going. A thorough process of strategic planning helps build team trust and pride. Executives need to listen to the heartbeat of the organization and look for opportunities to delegate planning responsibilities to those who will be responsible for implementing the plans.

As the confidence level builds in the organization because employees are listened to and respected, the staff will begin to participate in the creation of the future and will be more willing to grasp the need for change. In the health services field, much attention is paid to organizing systems that make it possible for the staff to provide the highest level of service to the individual patient. The direct providers of care are in the best position to provide input about organizational obstacles and changes that are needed to improve service. Not only do staff members need to be involved in the process of continually improving quality, but the patient—the beneficiary of the services—should also be involved. The system as a whole must move forward in this process to allow the kind of transformational change that is needed in the organization.

The CEO will also have the responsibility for watching out for barriers that are thrown up by individuals who feel more comfortable with the status quo than with the implementation of change. Individuals with more tenure or staff members with low energy levels may feel threatened by the possibility of new or different responsibilities, and therefore might be reluctant to be part of the planning process. The CEO needs to contain these barriers so that the process itself is not impaired.

Strategic planning is a commitment to organizational integration. Planning strategies are determined by the characteristics of an individual organization, the style of the leadership, the environmental needs, and the extent of the crises being faced. The challenge in the strategic planning process is to turn a vision into action and to do it in a fashion that permits as many people in the organization as possible to relate to that vision. The goals are to encourage involvement, to build the vision, and not to overdirect the details but to signal the general direction.

Conclusion

In recent years, Japanese and German industries have learned about the importance of an enterprising spirit. Their gains have been the result of a combination of vision and practical and rapid responses to change. Conversely, our industry has frequently been locked in traditional, long-range planning processes that have prevented rapid changes in direction. Now that we are accepting flexible, change-oriented approaches to planning, health care executives interested in ensuring the viability of their organizations can study these planning trends and work to understand change as the key to strategic planning.

Notes

1. R. H. Hayes, "Strategic Planning—Forward in Reverse," *Harvard Business Review* 63, no. 6 (1985): 114.
2. J. A. Byrne, "How the Best Get Better—Robert Waterman and His New Book, *The Renewal Factor*," *Business Week*, 14 September 1987.

PART III

FLEXIBILITY: ADAPTING TO
TURBULENT TIMES

8

CORPORATE RESTRUCTURING: DEALING WITH CHANGE AT THE MANAGEMENT LEVEL

Case in Point

In 1920, the founders of what is now known as the Virginia Mason Medical Center in Seattle created a single for-profit hospital and clinic. In 1934, the structure was changed and the hospital was separated into a nonprofit hospital (Virginia Mason Hospital) and a group practice that operated as a for-profit clinic (the Mason Clinic).

This structure worked well for the organization as it grew from its modest beginnings into a 200-physician group practice closely associated with the 320-bed Virginia Mason Hospital. In the 1950s, a nonprofit research component was incorporated, and in the early 1970s still another nonprofit structure (the Virginia Mason Foundation) was incorporated to solicit funds for the hospital and the research center.

Much of the high-tech equipment (radiology and other diagnostic services) was located in the clinic, and most of the hospital's professional services were provided by the staff of the clinic. The clinic's professional staff, as partners, contributed each year to the hospital and research center and also provided many functions of professional supervision at no charge to the hospital and research center.

When the clinic experienced a good month financially, the partners took more home. When times were not so good, their compensation dropped. When new equipment or new buildings were needed, the partnership acted on the need and funded the additions out of their own pockets. As the years rolled by, the assets of the partners grew, as did the amount of money required for new partners to buy their share of the asset base. When partners left the clinic, their shares were purchased by the partnership at book value.

By the mid-1980s, the clinic, hospital, and research center were all prospering. The total organization was on a growth curve that consumed increasing amounts of capital. It was essential, for example, that new primary practice sites be added to the system, but each additional satellite was capital intensive in its start-up phase.

The physicians and lay leaders in the leadership group felt that the time had arrived to design a major new structure to prepare for even further growth and contend with the competition brewing in the region. Further restructuring was needed to protect the organization's mission to provide medical education, research, and charity care. More capital was needed to provide for system growth, and a more stable base was required to handle the potentially volatile partnership financial issues.

Following a three-year process of study, a highly complex restructuring process was initiated that resulted in a new parent corporation (the Virginia Mason Medical Center), a new nonprofit subsidiary (the Virginia Mason Clinic), a second subsidiary (the Virginia Mason Hospital), and a third subsidiary (the Virginia Mason Research Center). In addition, the process folded the Virginia Mason Foundation into the new parent corporation and eliminated its separate nonprofit structure.

The plan required a complex approval process, which included passage of special state legislation to permit the practice of medicine by a nonprofit professional corporation (previously not permitted); acceptance of the new structure by the Internal Revenue Service; a vote within the clinic partnership (to approve the process); negotiation of the price for the purchase of all partnership assets by the new clinic organization from the partnership; the reconciliation of benefit programs; and a host of other conversion requirements.

Yet when the final vote of the clinic partnership took place, all but one of the partners voted for the conversion to the new structure. The one dissenter said he only voted in opposition to the transaction because he could "never tolerate any situation where the partners were unanimous"!

Life used to be simpler. Just as physicians these days must be frustrated with trying to keep up with technological changes, so are health care executives stressed by the speed of change in the delivery of services. To survive as executives in our volatile and competitive world, we learn quickly to be perpetual optimists. So when we contemplate the idea of restructuring, we think of it as an expression of accomplishment, as a sign of growth, and as a means of achieving new and higher levels of performance.

But if you really look at the word, you see that *re*-structuring implies responding to forces that demand change, which probably means contending or coping with some underlying challenges to the organization. Restructuring implies change, and change involves a risk to the status quo, and these risks invariably affect management.

Why Restructure?

Organizations restructure for a number of reasons. They restructure to raise capital, to improve the economy of scale or operational effectiveness, or to increase market share. They merge to increase competitive positions, to shield organizational assets from intervention. Restructuring is not usually driven by a single objective. Rather, it tends to occur when an organization faces a multitude of internal or external challenges.

The comments in this chapter will be applicable to a range of restructuring endeavors and models, including the creation of a new parent holding company controlling two operating subsidiaries that previously were independent organizations; the acquisition of one entity by another through a buy-out; a merger between two equal or unequal parties; the division of a single entity into new or additional operating components through a decentralization strategy; and the creation of binding affiliation or alliance agreements between two or more parties.

As an example, let's look at one single structure—the parent holding company—and examine the potential reasons for restructuring. We will assume that two independent but related health care organizations agree to place themselves under the operational control of a new parent holding company. The assets of the subsidiaries are taken under the control of the parent corporation, and the two entities function as an obligated group when raising capital and servicing debt. The new parent corporation possesses all of the typical reserve powers of any parent corporation, including budget control; ratification of the election of the subsidiary board, officers, and directors; control of bylaw changes; and approval of debt and sale or transfer of assets. The objectives for restructuring are to gain access to additional capital for growth, to strengthen market position by creating a single corporate image, and to achieve new economies of scale with a reduction of duplication of effort and activities.

The Impact on Management

The magnitude of the impact of restructuring on management correlates directly with the degree of shift in control from one unit to another. The corporate merger of two community hospitals, for example, has a much more profound impact on management than does the enrollment of a community hospital in a regional purchasing program. Mergers have the most profound effect on the management structure, since old competitors do not necessarily marry easily under a new corporate label. Leadership styles may be incompatible, and even the selection of an existing leader to head the new corporate structure causes tension between managers of the organizations. The tension is then quickly passed on to all levels of both organizations. The need to integrate benefit schedules to ensure equity for all joint employees carries serious implications (or at least the perception thereof) for job security. And it is not just management and employees who are affected. Boards are reconstituted and key roles are shared. Personal and professional egos come into conflict, making the courtship long and sometimes painful. Even sharing services can create tensions throughout the newly joined organizations.

The Role of Management: How Can Leaders Help?

Effective leadership is essential when preparing organizations for restructuring. Although the process of restructuring is not entirely within the leader's control, the leader can profoundly influence the outcome. Monitoring the internal and external environments provides insight into both the need for and the best timing for restructuring. In addition, communication with medical staff, board members, and employees sets the stage for change. The leader's ability to plan and consult with others will certainly contribute to the development of the process. But significant change is not driven solely by the CEO; all stakeholders will need to be involved. The CEO's role is to recognize the need for change, raise the stakeholders' awareness of that need, and then work to successfully orchestrate the process. Leadership involvement in the following three activities is essential to ensuring the success of the restructuring effort.

Developing a Vision

Long before the new structure is established, it is important to look at the big picture. You cannot expect people to climb aboard a train if you have not told them where they are going, so you will need a clearly articulated goal, a vision of the future. Creating an organizational vision requires involvement. You cannot just lay visions on top of folks; you must facilitate the creation of the vision so that it ultimately becomes part of the organization. And you hope that by being involved in the creation of the vision, everyone will buy into a common goal.

Designing the Structure

The design of the structure is affected by a number of variables such as how to make the structure function to meet predetermined objectives or goals, and how to address human resources needs. Do you design the structure first and find people to fit it, or do you design the structure around an existing staff? To make this point more meaningful, let's take the example of the parent holding company model and create a corporate headquarters with a chief executive officer. We will also add a chief financial officer to coordinate the financial activities of the two primary subsidiaries. While we are at it, we obviously need to add a nursing administrator at the corporate level to coordinate the nursing operations of the two operating subsidiaries. Of course, we will also need a corporate human resources director to coordinate and standardize all our human resources policies (benefits and so on). Our new model has simply added overhead, because the operating subsidiaries still need chief operating officers, nursing directors, financial officers, and others. At least this is what happens if nature takes its course.

To avoid much of this organizational bloating, people have to cooperate between entities, and this does not occur easily. It is not easy to design new structures because the impact on existing managers is so significant.[1] Early in the process the scale and size of the new structure must be defined, and careful consideration must be given to the predictable and usually eloquent arguments that will be used both to attempt to preserve the status quo within the subsidiary units and to broaden the staff to increase control at the parent level. It is important to monitor bureaucracy very carefully in this process.

Most decisions, particularly in closely related organizations, should continue to be made within subsidiary operating units. This creates a healthier, more responsive organization than one in which the corporate staff is large, controlling, and out of touch with or uninformed about what really goes on.[2] Corporate staff play a vital role in addressing policy and major program issues, and they need to tune in closely to subsidiary activities, monitoring events and offering counseling. But operating decisions are usually best made within the management structure of the local unit.

In designing new structures, keep in mind one note of caution. The process of decentralization requires competency at the level of the operating unit. In designing the structure you will be well advised to evaluate the staff to ensure that they can carry off their responsibilities and will cooperate with their counterparts in sister organizations. If your goal is to function with a lean corporate staff, you need to anticipate how specific corporate-related functions will be conducted.

Dealing with Uncertainty

As organizations go through change, it is always difficult to forecast the outcome with complete accuracy. You can create a plan, but you should anticipate the need for some mid-course adjustments. New organizations may go through several stages before the new structure finally settles down.

First, new structures go through a shakedown period in which governance and management processes are tested to determine how the new model works. This is a honeymoon stage in which leaders are given a chance to perform without considerable risk. However, it is not without stress, since leaders know that the honeymoon stage will not last forever.

Once the honeymoon stage is over, a process of fine-tuning takes place. Assumptions and predictions made during the planning stage are reviewed. New financial forecasts are made. The cultures of the newly joined organizations are usually shocked when new team leaders begin to exert their authority over team members who were used to a different approach. In addition, some steps initially taken to make the merger or restructuring possible will have to be renegotiated as the dust begins to settle and confidence in the new structure begins to build. For example, if the combined board of two newly merged hospitals proves to be too large to be effective, it may have to be reduced gradually through rotation over the next few years.

The point in referring to these stages of change is that the new structures will not mature if operating formats are locked up too quickly. Just as in buying a new set of clothes, some tailoring is usually required. Management must build enough credibility to be able to initiate further change and to overcome any resistance they might encounter in staff who are affected by the process. Senior executives who are leading the restructuring process need to protect their credibility, be highly visible during the process, and conserve their reserves so that they have enough energy and resources when it comes time to address the second or, in some cases, the third stage of the process.

The Ten Essentials for Survival

The leadership role in the restructuring process will be most significant if the leader is able to work with the following points in mind. Following these guidelines will help to minimize the trauma to all in the organization during periods of restructuring.

1. *Never underestimate the amount of personal energy required to carry off the new structure.* Personal energy is a depletable resource. The impact of change is substantial, and when you are attempting to lead a process, it means being on point for extended periods of time. Burnout is possible at any level in new structures, so the executive has a responsibility not only to monitor his or her own energy but also to protect the energy levels of others who are critical to the process.

2. *Keep a close eye on the external environment.* The process of restructuring has a tendency to blind key leaders because their attention is so inwardly focused. The executive investing heavily in the future may fail to spot significant external trends that will affect the organization. For example, a leader in a single unit might work diligently on internal restructuring but fail to fully appreciate the extent of the accumulated losses beginning to build in capitated plans throughout a region. This might translate into unexpected provider discounts and a fall in revenue at home. By failing to monitor this external factor, the executive could experience an unexpected capital "bleed" (an executive's nightmare in which cash flow reaches the critical "red line" and institutional bankers begin to monitor, limit, or reduce the organization's credit line).

3. *Continually track actual progress against reorganization or restructuring feasibility plans.* The typical organization undergoing restructuring develops thorough feasibility plans that include detailed forecasts of volume and revenue. Once restructuring has been implemented, there may be a tendency to ignore deviations from the original plan. This is usually a mistake. The feasibility plan marks the path toward certain goals; it provides a measuring stick for determining whether the goals are actually being met. Variances between actual and predicted operating plans need analysis to allow timely mid-course adjustments.

4. *Control the organization's capital.* One reason for pursuing restructuring is that it might enhance the acquisition of new capital. Although the usual decision-making constraints with respect to allocation of new capital are still in place, the enthusiasm and optimism associated with restructuring sometimes leads to short-range decisions that will haunt the organization at a later time. New capital is often spent too easily. Leaders would be wise to put a tight cap on expenditures. There will almost certainly be some surprises along the way that will consume capital at an alarming rate.

5. *Increase team-building activities.* Communication problems increase in geometric proportions in larger, more complicated structures. Organizations that elect to create a separate corporate headquarters will find that this complicates communications and makes it more difficult to build integrated managment teams. Executives need to anticipate this and intensify the development of additional communication methods (retreats, enhanced publications, reassessment of committee and meeting structures, and so on).

6. *Keep governing boards fully informed and involved.* Returning to our parent holding company model, which would most typically create a new parent board, care has to be taken to ensure that trustees can make the transition from an operating board environment to a board that deals more with policy and reserve powers. The orientation and educational processes for board members have to be accelerated.

7. *Involve the medical staff.* If the new structure is going to flourish, physicians need to be involved early in the planning process and encouraged to participate throughout. Executives who do not encourage physician involvement should not be surprised at a less than enthusiastic response to major change. Executives need to motivate, encourage, and reward involved members of their medical staff. Physicians are needed both to help develop the vision and to participate in implementing change.

8. *Guard against "group think."* If clear signals are given from the top that input is not welcome, an unhealthy set of circumstances will surface. Team members begin to draw back, perhaps to protect their turf, and a group think process takes place in which no one feels free to voice their opinion. When management assignments are changed, job boundaries often become blurred, and in the reshuffling there is always the possibility that team members who are facing uncertainty will feel safer simply agreeing with suggestions than expressing their honest opinions. The leader must obtain decision-making input without depending too much on consensus building, but also without taking a single-handed approach. It is a task that calls for patience and a balanced approach.

9. *Seek new ways to reward innovation.* When undergoing restructuring there is a tendency to rely on customary practices to resolve new challenges. While this works in many cases, overreliance on traditional methods and procedures may make it difficult for the organization to make necessary decisions. It is very difficult to dismantle approaches that have worked comfortably in the past

and to adopt new tools and techniques that are unfamiliar. But executives need to recognize the hazard of overreliance on familiar practices and must lead the way by being innovative. This is where the *art* of leadership surfaces. A positive attitude toward change has to be conveyed throughout the organization.[3] If somebody in the organization attempts to block change (saying, for example, "we've tried it before and it doesn't work"), executives should move quickly to reverse the attitude (for example, by responding that "it may not have worked in the past, but this is a good time to try it again"). Those members of the staff who are willing to and capable of change should always be appropriately and publicly recognized and rewarded.

10. *Devote enough time to thinking.* "Thinking time" tends to evaporate in the face of constant change. As new relationships are established within the organization, it is important to reflect on how things are proceeding and why they are unfolding as they are. If a colleague begins to function in an unpredictable fashion in the new structural setting, spend some time thinking through the reasons for the behavior so that you can respond thoughtfully and effectively. This type of reflection is critical to a successful outcome. It helps the executive to make mid-course adjustments, altering the plan or recommending special counseling to find an early resolution if there is a problem. Executives responsible for the change process must protect enough time to isolate themselves and reflect on some of the more subtle dynamics that may be occurring in the organization.

Conclusion

Restructuring has significant and unpredictable effects on management. Some health care executives and managers, particularly older executives who have built their careers on a different set of conditions, will be unable to accept the level of change required. Successful restructuring requires time and energy, and one should expect some unexpected and painful experiences before the whole process is complete.

Do not underestimate the amount of insecurity, resistance, and criticism you may encounter in all participants, including subsidiary board members, medical staff, management, members of the community who previously identified with one entity or another, and employees at all levels. Each constituency group needs to be assessed to measure its level of understanding of the process. Misunderstanding and resistance should be recognized early, and plans to modify attitudes should be implemented quickly to improve the odds of success. New relationships can and often do create testy and difficult situations. The wise executive pays close attention to the task at hand and monitors events very closely during such times.

Notes

1. J. Flower, "The Role of the Leader," *Healthcare Forum* 33, no. 3 (1990): 30–34.
2. D. Burda, "Untangling Management Structures," *Modern Healthcare* 20, no. 17 (1990): 25–28.
3. S. Berger and S. Sudman, "Merging Cultures: Successful CEOs Read Warning Signs," *Healthcare Executive* 5, no. 2 (1990): 21–23.

9

PREPARING FOR STRATEGIC INTEGRATION

Case in Point

Some time ago, a colleague of mine in California received a telephone call from an administrator of a neighboring hospital who wanted to discuss the possibility of a merger. It was a straightforward suggestion based on a mutual problem. The proposal was intended to address the possibility that neither hospital alone could survive the impending health system changes but that together both might survive.

Over the years, both operations had grown and prospered. One was hospital oriented, with small group practices and a staff of solo practitioners. This hospital had newer buildings and lots of cash. The other operation had an older hospital structure, but it included a large multispecialty group practice that was tightly integrated with the hospital. This organization also had a prospering primary care network of ten clinics. Because it had invested heavily in the future, its capital was less readily available.

My colleague's neighbor retained a consultant who was convinced that a merger of the two organizations would be an ideal arrangement for both parties. But when the two administrators started negotiating, several major problems surfaced, making the success of such a venture seem highly unlikely.

The basic proposal called for the relocation of the large group practice to the neighbor's site. But this would have meant breaking up a model that was already well positioned for the future—a highly integrated hospital-based group practice focusing on the growth and integration of ambulatory services. The proposal also seemed to ignore the many problems associated with merging medical staffs (competition for operating room times, decisions on the provision of diagnostic services previously provided by the group practice, antitrust questions, and a multitude of other issues). Neither organization would be able to operate without attending to the needs and activities of its own staff members.

Discussions between the parties finally ended on a positive note. There were services that could be shared and programs that could be developed on a cooperative basis or through a joint venture. But a merger was out of the question at this point, particularly without a good deal more trust between the principals. The proposed merger appeared to some as more of a competitive takeover than a merger: "Give us your medical staff, abandon your hospital, and all will be well."

The process of working out the terms of the merger and preparing for strategic integration would require an incredible commitment of time and energy on the part of both executives. The executives realized that before they would be willing to undertake such a commitment, they would have to demonstrate not only that a merger would offer achievable cost efficiencies and improved quality but that the missions and cultures of the two organizations could somehow be reconciled. If the stakes changed later and the two organizations had to reconsider a merger as a means of economic survival, at least then they would know where to start.

Organizations are never still; they always seem to be gathering momentum, either growing and expanding or gradually coming apart. Once the momentum starts, it may be very difficult for some organizations to change their direction, so building relationships with other organizations may be the only way for them to resist the changes that threaten to bring about their demise. Excellent leadership throughout the process of strategic integration can make the difference in determining whether or not the organization can begin to grow again under a new structure.

Throughout the next decade, with more and more health care decisions made under the pressure of organizational instability and rapid change, we will learn more and more about ourselves as leaders and about our organizations. Strategic integration will demand excellent leadership, and leaders will be required to sustain the rigor, wisdom, and vision necessary to foster the process.

Rationale for Integration: Why Merge or Link?

Environmental Preconditions

In early 1988, the Harris Poll suggested that almost 89 percent of Americans believed that the U.S. health care system needed fundamental change.[1] The alleged dissatisfaction with the status quo is just one of many complex dynamics in today's health care arena. This is an era filled with contrasts, including tremendous and growing disparity in access to and dissemination of funds and services.

Although the conflicting demands in health care are in part reflective of larger societal issues, the health care environment consists of a number of unique conditions that have made the survival of some health care organizations tenuous at best. Most struggling health care organizations are dealing with one or more of three types of circumstances. First, there are conditions over which the organization has little if any control, such as the federal government decision to freeze physician payments at the 1984 fee level. Another example is the decision made by a major employer to move 90,000 employees from an indemnity market health insurance product into a closed-panel managed care system, which excludes a great number of provider hospitals that previously provided hospital services to those employees and their families.

Second, there are conditions that the organization should have predicted but did not, as in the case of a skilled nursing facility that fails to watch its payer mix and ends up in financial default because of poor forecasting. Similarly, if an organization (perhaps a hospital) knows that a neighboring institution with a heavy Medicaid population is floundering, it *ought* to prepare for an influx of additional charity and Medicaid patients. Another example is a decision to open a new medical service without adequately researching the competitive environment; research might have revealed that the project was doomed because of late entry into the market.

Third, some environmental conditions are caused by the organization itself. A hospital that sponsors the development of a primary care group practice but in the process alienates its medical staff (who in turn retaliate by moving their patients to a competing hospital) has created a hostile atmosphere for itself. A similar situation occurs when lack of direction from the board freezes the ability of management to make decisions and prevents the organization from taking advantage of opportunities. Finally, if a popular and effective administrator simply loses the ability to lead, and no one in the organization is willing to confront this in a timely fashion, the organization will gradually lose its credibility.

Motivating Factors

Depending on the severity of the environmental circumstances affecting the organization's operation, the organization may be in a position of needing to undertake some kind of strategic integration attempt to bring itself out of the debilitating situation. Leaders in any organization tend to merge or link with others for one or more of four reasons.

First, the organization's mission statement is sometimes a compelling motivator. The hospital or health care institution with a clearly defined mission of providing charity care might seek linkages with community clinics to make it possible for those clinics to survive. A hospital group with a religious mission could embark on an acquisition program that would never be undertaken in the absence of that mission. In these situations, the mission justifies greater risks than might otherwise be the case.

Second, an organization might wish to increase its competitive advantage (e.g., by merging with or buying out a competitor in order to provide a full range of services in the years ahead). A suburban hospital, for example, might merge with a much smaller hospital and then convert it into a skilled nursing facility to allow centralized acute care services with a linked but controlled skilled nursing capacity. Obviously, there might be antitrust issues to consider, but the point is that the merger provides a pretty good match for the two organizations' needs.

Third, the desire to strengthen the organization's financial security sometimes leads to a merger or linkage with another organization. A hospital might acquire adjacent residential apartment buildings and operate them profitably to add to the financial security of the parent organization. Similarly, a medical group practice that acquires a company providing mobile x-ray service to nursing homes and skilled nursing facilities adds to its financial security by vertically integrating related health services. Financial security is, of course, related to mission, competitive advantage, and other factors; likewise, diversification strategies are tightly linked to the goal of reinforcing the organization's financial security. (A decision to link with a national multi-institutional program might result from the need for access to resources to improve the organization's market share, or from a desire to link with a system to enhance its local image).

Finally, concern over the institution's image (or, at times, the CEO's ego) can result in a perceived need for strategic integration. Some leaders take inordinate pride in organizational size, and they may decide to merge or link organizations to increase facility capacity beyond what is reasonable. If this drive for a high organizational profile produces the desired results, the shear power of the larger organization will force weaker competitors to pay attention. If the increased capacity does not work, there will probably be a change in management.

Successful Integration: Leadership Priorities

What conditions aid the organization as it struggles through decisions relating to integration and linking? Conditions will vary depending on the organization, but the most influential conditions are the outgrowth of effective leadership. Leaders who wish to have the greatest impact on integration should concentrate on a number of specific areas before the organization will be ready for and capable of strategic integration.

The Mission

A clearly understood and articulated organizational mission, against which new ventures can be compared and considered, is absolutely critical to successful strategic integration. An organization without an understood mission is unfocused, operating with seemingly accidental decision-making processes and achieving interesting but unplanned and unpredictable results. Haphazard diversification, for example, can lead to overextended resources. Linking and diversification strategies should relate clearly to the organization's main mission, and an organization with a strong leader will ensure that that mission is focused and well defined.[2] The leader's role is not only to see that the organization's mission statement is highly visible and that new programs relate to the mission but also to serve as a monitor to ensure that the mission is scrutinized so that it reflects the organization's values and direction.

Capital and Human Resources

The amount of financial and human capital available will be influential in determining the success of a strategic integration attempt. Success may be achieved by using accumulated capital to acquire or link with others to further increase economies of scale and market presence. Weaker organizations might strengthen their positions by linking with larger, more competitive organizations in order to gain access to resources. Although this is an area over which the organization's leader may not have total control, he or she will want to encourage decision making within the organization that reinforces the most effective use of resources. The secret to successful investment of capital and human resources in the integration process is making sure that the linkage has something in it for both parties.

Leadership Continuity

Although most people acknowledge the importance of competent and credibile leadership in creating an environment that lends itself to linkages, the importance of continuity is often overlooked. The turnover rate among hospital chief executives is now running at about 18 to 20 percent per year. This is especially disturbing when we consider the time it takes to build responsive management teams (three to five years) and to start organizations moving down the right path. Although turnover can sometimes be a sign that the organization is working on building its team, continual turnover is destructive and usually indicates that the organization is being subjected to constant changes in direction without any rallying point.

A new CEO usually initiates new practices. The new CEO is probably being brought in to correct problems and to change the organization's course of direction (although this may not be the case when an executive retires and succession planning has occurred). Organizations that have learned how to bring new leaders into existing structures without disrupting daily operations are usually most effective at building successful and continuing management practices.

Rapid, sudden swings in any new direction, especially if they consume vast quantities of financial and human capital, increase risks and make the outcome of integration less predictable. A certain amount of predictability will contribute to prospective partners' confidence in the organization's leadership. Solid performance and advancement, combined with a clearly understood philosophy of incremental growth, stabilizes the organization and permits it to grow.

In times of instability, caution is usually the key. Instability may result from financial losses, excessive employee or medical staff turnover, the board's lack of trust in the CEO's decision-making abilities, or any number of other factors in the organization. The leader must assess risks carefully. On the other hand, it is important to guard against the kind of stagnation that results from being frozen by the fear of taking risks, and to be willing to make decisions that will carry the organization forward.

Conflict Resolution

In any change-oriented environment, conflict is inevitable. Mechanisms for diffusing internal conflict need to be in place to maximize the opportunity to link with others. Merging organizations will probably be battered when their missions, cultures, and management styles begin to collide. Evidence of this clash is found in the tendency of CEOs of one or both of two merged organizations to relocate soon after the integration process has been completed. Leaders who want to be involved in successful partnerships with other organizations should plan for these inevitable conflicts by addressing issues such as board involvement and oversight, management interchange, and the impact the merger will have on the culture and climate of the new structure.

Optimism and an Enterprising Attitude

Organizations must retain leaders who recognize the virtues of optimism and an enterprising attitude. Leaders at all levels in the organization need to consider whether, as the saying goes, the glass is half full or half empty. The answer to this question reveals a lot about the strategy that will be employed during these times. The executive who has just endured the burden of downsizing an organization to improve its financial condition, and who then promotes the development of a new service that may have to be subsidized for a year or two, sends a compelling message to the staff. Some may perceive the action as an indication that the leader is out of control. After all, why invest in the future while at the same time cutting back? A more optimistic interpretation, however, is that the worst is over and the organization is on the move again. It is up to the leader to present the strategy in a way that carries the desired message to the staff.

Where to Start

In preparing organizations for integration, there are a number of specific things the leader can do to influence the process. First, leaders should work to reconcile differences in management style. It is difficult enough to do this in a single institutional setting, but in interinstitutional relationships where there is likely to be competition for turf (as is common in full integration), leaders can expect turmoil. Reconciliation of management style differences takes time and must be based on trust and interdependence. Without trust between the principals the integration attempt (and the individuals involved) might be doomed to failure.

Try to develop a consensus of understanding about the combined mission of the newly integrated organization. When missions of different organizations are merged, they may appear similar, but the cultural background of each of the integrating organizations may not be as similar as initially perceived. For example, the integration of an urban tertiary care center and a newly acquired primary care satellite group, which is somewhat distant from the urban center, sounds like "a natural" in that patients who need specialty care will be referred downtown and patients who need primary care will be referred to the suburban satellite. But physicians like to follow patients, and patients like to follow physicians. So some patients who could have been referred to the downtown tertiary center will still be admitted to a local hospital because it is easier for the primary physician to follow the patient there than it would be to follow the patient downtown. The dynamics become increasingly complex as linkages and integration efforts are implemented. The challenge is to create an awareness and understanding of the big picture and thereby to skillfully increase motivation.

The leader addresses this kind of problem by first identifying the issues. In the above example, exactly what is the magnitude of the problem? Has the organization contributed to the issue through failing to define expectations? The involved parties must be consulted so that consensus can be reached. Solutions are then developed and monitoring processes are installed to measure progress.

It is essential that the leader recognize the amount of time that will be needed to resolve such an issue. Problems affecting attitudes often require the most time for resolution. Of course, ultimately the focus should always be on what is best for the patient.

Yet another management challenge is the transfer of management skills when a cohesive leadership group in a single environment suddenly must take on new operational programs. For example, when a hospital acquires a durable medical equipment company and decides that management styles need to be integrated to achieve maximum results, an endless list of questions and issues are raised. Can a manager from the core organization apply skills in a specialty subdivision? Can the human resources director attract applicants for diverse structures? Will the information systems division be able to establish communication and linkages related to financial data in order to assist in the integration of the organizations, or will the division impose an impossible bureaucracy on the smaller units?

Increased organizational size inevitably leads to increased bureaucracy, and even a benevolent bureaucracy will be perceived as a threat by those being absorbed into a larger organization. Large organizations are more difficult to manage than small organizations, simply because the number of people involved changes the pace and challenges the ability of leaders to manage processes.

Finally, the leader of a large integrated structure must maintain the values of the old system in spite of the new growth. This may require changes in management style or the investment of resources and education to develop new communication systems at different levels in the organization. Organizations may need to flatten hierarchical structures so that more people are involved in decision making at the lowest possible level in the organization, thereby driving decision making from the bottom rather than from the top.

New structures born of vertical or horizontal integration experience massive changes. Because bureaucracy in enlarged organizations becomes especially complex, leaders must be willing to accept the significant challenge of managing bureaucratic systems.

What to Avoid

There are probably more things guaranteed to go wrong than to go right in the process of overseeing strategic integration. A number of common mistakes made by leaders who wrestle with the operational aspects of integration can be avoided. Leaders who want to ensure a successful merger or linkage should be wary of the following potentially disastrous circumstances.

Undercapitalization

Leaders who undertake new ventures are often surprised by how quickly capital and cash can flow in the wrong direction. Too frequently, managerial optimism takes over, and once the venture is underway there are a thousand reasons why "all it needs is a little more time."

The decision to continue is often directly related to the chain of command. The president's idea is likely to be given more time to succeed than an idea that comes from down the line, and the organization will be much more sensitive in putting the president's venture to the acid test of financial reality. Failure to appreciate the potency of the power at the top can contribute to the failure of the project, and failure to implement backup measures can lead to financial disaster.

Several years ago, a midwestern community with two hospitals was trying to address the fact that it could really only support one hospital. The administrator of the weaker hospital would not accept the need for a merger. As a result, the hospital operated with a deficit year after year until it was no longer viable. Virtually everyone in the community knew that as each year passed the negotiating power of the organization was weakened, but because of the power of the CEO (and the weakness of the board), the inevitable was deferred until it was too late to salvage the operation. The hospital was finally sold to the other organization, but it was a distress sale. There was no room for negotiation because the CEO had let the opportunity slip away. The CEO's stubbornness and failure to acknowledge reality took its toll on the organization, its employees, and the community.

A similar situation in the business world occurred in Toledo, Ohio, where a local bank president truly believed that downtown Toledo could be revitalized. Indeed, under his direction it was revitalized . . . for a while.

But the financial planning was not solid, the bank was overextended, and ultimately all of the board and officers resigned. The bank president's enthusiasm and civic zeal blinded him to the reality of financial circumstances and brought the bank to its knees. Fail-safe and oversight mechanisms were not in place. The management team probably was not able to express a dissenting viewpoint because the organization's mission (to revitalize the community) was so pristine and the CEO's charisma must have caused them to put logic aside. In addition, the relative prosperity of the external environment probably made them feel fairly secure—at least initially—in following the CEO's lead.

Too Much Planning

We all talk about the need for solid long-range plans in health care organizations, and at the same time we expound the need for incremental planning. But there has to be a middle ground. High-risk ventures take more time to plan than low-risk ventures. Ventures requiring a high infusion of capital require more discussion and study than do those with low capital or cost impacts. Yet there must be a time to stop studying something and to start acting on it.

When confronted with the internal politics that play a crucial part in the process of strategic integration, the wise chief executive officer will try to keep a clear head and a little distance from the points of contention in order to steady the planning process. Freezing decision making until all points are absolutely nailed down, all risks are eliminated, and total consensus is achieved usually signals that the organization has become immobilized. By the time a decision is made in such an organization, the service or program may have been bypassed by its competition. Although it is important to proceed cautiously, the leader must recognize the time to act.

For example, a hospital's unexpected opportunity to purchase a mobile x-ray company, which serviced some 60 nursing homes, had to be assessed rapidly or the opportunity would be lost. The hospital had not previously identified such a service as a priority, but the project was determined to be viable and the decision to purchase was made on a faster track than usual. In this instance, the internal politics associated with "selling" a controversial project were absent. The project was an obvious "win/win situation" from the very beginning.

Ignoring the External Environment

Focusing on internal operations to the extent that you exclude careful environmental surveillance is another habit to avoid. When the staff casts about and tries to get ahead but at the same time ignores its competition, the organization is like a kingdom under seige. The moat is cleaned and stocked with crocodiles, the drawbridge is locked up tight, and all of the knights and soldiers guard the castle walls around the clock—all in anticipation of an enemy who may or may not appear over the next hill. Without any knowledge of the competing forces, even the best defense will only protect the kingdom and will not help the king get the advantage in the attack.

Decisions that deal only with problems within the confines of the castle are hazardous. Knowing your operation so that your organization can be proactive is essential, but this also means knowing your competitor and continuing to channel your organization's energy into innovative advances that allow it to adapt to environmental conditions. For example, integrated organizations that are to function in the context of and stay afloat with today's conditions will need data-based systems that can merge financial and clinical data in a way that is usable and cost-effective. These days health care leaders cannot afford to operate under siege conditions unless their bank accounts are very large. Mobility, external intelligence, adaptability, and movement are the directions for the day. Care must be taken to look at opportunities for strategic integration and to act on them when internal and external conditions are right.

Unwillingness to Divest

If the moment comes when you realize that the integration process is not going to work, it will take courage to deal with the implications. There are risks to admitting to a mistake, regardless of whether or not it is your responsibility.[3] Staff members might be worried about the future of their own jobs, their credibility in future endeavors, or their ability to take necessary risks in the future. Perhaps more likely, however, they find it difficult to acknowledge that their project simply did not succeed. Yet, in spite of their reluctance to let go of something that they helped create, there comes a time when the loss must be confronted, and the leader will have to address it with sensitivity and persistence.

Look for ways to help colleagues "save face." Sensitivity in these situations will pay off later when your associates recognize that appropriate risk taking is a virtue, not a handicap. Failure to acknowledge and allow the grieving of a lost project will suggest to staff, some of whom may be your most innovative thinkers, that you are indifferent about their efforts and the worth of the project. Leaders can facilitate the transition from losing to winning by admitting that a project has not succeeded while at the same time recognizing the efforts of those who participated in it.

Insufficient Staffing

Executives have been so bullied by issues of cost containment that they are sometimes inclined to reduce the very resources they need to cope successfully with the organization's integration. Leaders who become too absorbed in setting the example might fail to examine whether what they are doing is actually the best thing for the organization. Perhaps hospital executives believe that they must always be the first to cut staff or reduce travel if they expect managers and staff to reduce expenses elsewhere in the organization. Yet entire management staffs have been demoralized and destroyed by senior executives who have felt so compelled to lead the cost reduction charge that they did not realize they were doing away with the very resources that would make it possible for the organization to achieve its goals.

When times are tough, take time to reflect and consider what you are doing to the organization when you curtail the means by which the organization as a whole will be able to respond to changes and challenges. If you do not think through the processes carefully, you will find yourself trying to cope with an administrative style better suited to fire fighting, but without any fire trucks at a five-alarm fire. It takes foresight to protect the capacity of the organization to respond to change, and it also takes a good staff. But it takes years to turn around the culture and financial stability of an organization in which everyone's attention has been focused on the bottom line without consideration of the organization's mission.

The Politics of Indecision

Paralysis occurs when it becomes difficult to make decisions in a timely fashion because executives are bound to "management by total consensus." Because consensus means different things to different people, the executive is often in a position of needing to find a way to accommodate or overrule various decision-making perspectives. For example, consensus as defined by the autocrat occurs when everyone is silent on an issue; the lack of verbal input means that everyone agrees. The person who believes in complete democracy, however, sees consensus as a process in which everyone in the room has their say before their final votes are tallied. To the realist, consensus means something different still: that the issues have been discussed, the proper attention has been paid to the political factions involved, and a proposal is made to resolve the matter in a timely fashion.

The executive's leadership style is extremely important in determining how the plans for strategic integration get ironed out. Rather than working with the whole group to settle every issue on the spot, the leader sometimes needs to be able to listen, consider the issue in sufficient depth, and then act to resolve the problem and move on to the next plateau. The executive will be paralyzed without eventually drawing the benevolent politics of decision making to a close. A leader who is unwilling to take the risks inherent in decision making is likely to fall back on the much-used phrase, "We need more information."

Ignoring the Mission

If you really want to shake up an organization, outline a sensible proposal for strategic integration, define and articulate the mission, and then at the last minute, change the ground rules. Instead of proceeding with the merger or linkage, adopt a new product or program that is in direct conflict with the stated mission of the organization and then pour resources into the project. Here are a couple of examples of what might happen:

Midtown Health Network. Midtown Health Network, which has a clearly stated mission involving care of the aged, has been putting resources into geriatric programs, hiring additional specialists, and working on plans to develop a sophisticated program offering a full range of services for the elderly. Then suddenly the organization decides to focus on occupational medicine. The emphasis on care to the aged is diminished, and resources are redirected. The effect on middle management and others in the organization is such that no one knows what they should be doing.

Urban Health Plan. Urban Health Plan decides to purchase an outside printing company and expend the capital allotted for the purchase of high-tech equipment for patient services (the organization's main mission) on setting up the new venture. As a result, employees, physicians, and managers are completely confused about the direction the organization is taking. Their understandably frantic reaction is itself enough to slow down the organization's operations.

What does all this have to do with the pitfalls and perils of integration? The point is that there are unlimited opportunities to confuse the troops. Leaders who want to link and integrate should have their house in order, and that means respecting the organization's mission and counting on others to do the same.

Lack of Vision

When things begin to go awry, many executives become blind to reality and unable to accept difficult circumstances. They may become pessimistic, overlooking opportunities to turn things around and thereby contributing to the reality of the downward spiral—that is, the perception that conditions in the organization are so catastrophic that nothing can be done to make them better.

Capable leaders avoid being blinded under stressful conditions. They have achieved a certain level of professional maturity that allows them to lead, keeping the spirit of the organization up and still coping with the volatility of the health care environment. Organizations need visionary leaders to stay focused on the benefits and positive outcomes that strategic integration can produce. Leaders project out beyond the darkness and into a brighter future.

Preparing organizations for strategic integration is largely a matter of disseminating the leader's vision throughout the organization as a whole. Organizations that link successfully are usually characterized by leaders with a vision of what the organization could be and belief in the organization's ability to get there.

Inflated Ego

Although ego can be a motivating factor for integration and linkage, it can also contribute to the failure of essential strategies involved in the integration. There is nothing more damaging to the development of a good interinstitutional relationship than arrogance, whether real or perceived, on the part of either organization. Arrogance is a destructive factor that leads to the failure of many joint ventures.

Excessive ego ultimately translates into the destruction of an organization's capacity to respond to community or service needs. Inflated institutional or executive egos must be dealt with quickly and judiciously by health care boards and leaders. Linkages and ventures will not last if they are based on the threat and power associated with the assertion of a dominating individual or institution. Successful and lasting ventures are based on trust, reconciliation of mission, and good hard work at building interpersonal credibility and respect among the principals.

The Big Picture

Based on forecasts of consumer dissatisfaction, concerns about costs, and the other pressures being brought to bear on health care, we can expect that the field will continue to change dramatically over the next several years. The big picture for all of us depends on how well we as individuals are able to cope in this era of confusion and challenge. As we consider the need for strategic integration, we should develop an attitude toward and philosophy of leadership with a few basic ideas in mind:

1. *The importance of space and time.* It is very important for today's leader to find time to think, to reflect on the significance of events so as to carry out deliberate plans and responsibilities.

2. *The importance of learning by doing.* We establish our credibility by trying and succeeding at new things. Credibility makes the difference when you are trying to change the system.

3. *The need to avoid elitism.* Even the best leader cannot do it alone. Avoid isolation and build a structure that allows you to have comfortable access to information and to feel secure in others' decision-making abilities.

4. *The need to develop a management style.* Leaders must learn to modify their style based on need when strategic integration brings about a changing organizational life.

5. *The willingness to recognize personal shortcomings.* Leaders must continually assess strengths and weaknesses, and then develop additional strengths.

6. *The need to protect professional and personal integrity.* Nothing is more valuable if you believe that you can make a difference.

7. *The importance of knowing your limits.* Health administration is a tough field, and it is going to require considerable strength and dedication to meet the challenges and opportunities that will characterize the next ten to fifteen years. Do not be afraid to say you have had enough.

Conclusion

Organizational integration requires, first, that your house is in order, and second, that you have the resources to carry off the venture successfully. But the most important requirement is that you take the time to carefully and decisively determine where you want to end up. Reluctance to balance caution with a degree of opportunism suggests that either you will act precipitously or you will not act at all. Venturing into relationships with other organizations really is not very mysterious, especially if it is grounded in common sense. As in any lasting human relationship, a foundation of trust will prove to be beneficial to both parties.

Notes

1. M. Terris, "Lessons from Canada's Health Program," *Technology Review* 93 (February/March 1990): 26–33.
2. S. M. Shortell, E. Morrison, and S. Hughes, "The Keys to Successful Diversification: Lessons from Leading Hospital Systems," *Hospital & Health Services Administration* 34, no. 4 (1989): 471–92.
3. J. Goldsmith, "The Hospital as We Know It Is Too Costly, Too Unwieldy, and Too Inflexible to Survive: A Radical Prescription for Hospitals," *Harvard Business Review* 67, no. 3 (1989): 104–11.

10

ORGANIZATIONAL LINKAGES: WORKING OUT THE NEW RELATIONSHIP

Case in Point

The Health Services Consortium in western Washington is a group of linked organizations that has operated to the benefit of all of its participating organizations since its inception in 1972. In 1991, the consortium had grown to a membership of 18 hospitals, ranging in size from 16 to 320 beds. It is a rural-urban linkage, and all of the members are independently governed. Members include traditional not-for-profit community hospitals, district (government-owned) hospitals, and several hospitals in a religious chain.

The consortium employs a full-time staff and is directed by a steering committee of administrators and representatives from each of the participating units. Each hospital, regardless of its size, has one vote on the committee. Member hospitals are obligated only to pay dues, and they can select offered programs without obligation. The program includes central purchasing and other similar activities, a strong component of medical education (offered on-site in the rural communities), and sophisticated linking of supervisors and others (through formal workshops) to encourage the continual exchange of operational information. Board members, medical staff members, and the members of the management team of each institution are involved not only in setting program goals but in the monitoring and evaluation of results.

Adapted from Austin Ross, "Organizational Linkages: Management Issues and Implications," *Hospital & Health Services Administration* 26, no. 2 (1981): 37–49.

The Health Services Consortium is not an incorporated body. Its existence is based on a principle of goodwill and a focus on programs relating to the missions of the individual hospitals. For years, observers have predicted its demise because so many other voluntary shared projects between hospitals have failed. Yet the consortium flourishes even in the absence of bylaws and a highly visible corporate structure. The model is at the opposite end of the organizational spectrum from the corporate hospital chain. Yet the principles of good management apply regardless of the difference in control and ownership.

The linking of complex health care organizations has tremendous potential for affecting both the quality and the cost of health care. In recent times, the rate of growth of linked arrangements has been comparable to the Oklahoma land rush. Linking seems to be popular almost everywhere, and it is fascinating to observe the development of linked organizations. Today, organizations concentrate on linkages between hospitals; but in the years ahead, relationships will be common between hospitals and related group practices, between nursing homes and home care agencies, and between other varieties of health services facilities.

A number of these relationships have developed because of the introduction of competition into health services. Evidence of new marketplace forces may be found in the growth of privately sponsored health maintenance organizations as well as in more traditional fee-oriented health services. A healthy dose of free enterprise has surfaced in a field that had been virtually written off by health economists as one dominated by noncompetitive, isolated units providing inefficient services, enveloped in medical politics, and operating in an environment where traditional principles of supply and demand were inapplicable.

Successfully linked models seem to develop somewhat independently, almost as if a germ of the idea was planted in different areas of the country and adapted to local conditions. A rich mixture of incentives contributes to their growth and success. There is a financial incentive to increase profitability by increasing volume and improving the economy of scale. There is the age-old need to market services to protect or improve patient referrals. Survival incentives are particularly popular with centrally located urban hospitals that face competition from the growth in suburban medical facilities. Some institutions respond to an incentive to serve rural populations, which stimulates growth and linkages between urban and rural physicians.

A common thread in many successful models is the matching of executive leadership with an environment of institutional expansion and solvency. Often these organizational relationships do not develop according to any carefully prepared long-range plan. Instead, they seem to grow in response to short-range concerns coupled with the ability of those involved to recognize opportunities. At each critical point in the model's development it seems that leaders are present who understand the need to take risks. And because the institution is in the position of wanting and probably needing to expand, the leaders are able to act on their impulses.

Vertical versus Horizontal Integration

A vertically or horizontally integrated organization is a group of institutions that share a common set of goals, some resources and management, and service to a common, specific population, one not necesssarily limited or defined by geography. These organizations need not be under common ownership, although the more they are integrated, the more likely they are to operate under single ownership, integrated management, and a common medical staff. These three features make it easier to achieve the critical mass necessary to control and manage change.

The difference between a vertically integrated structure and a horizontally integrated structure is in the service mix. In a vertically integrated structure, the patient moves within the system to receive the treatment needed. For example, the patient in a rural hospital is transferred to a central institution for specialty services. Thereafter, the patient is returned to a community hospital or a community home care agency for continuing services. All services are linked within one organizational framework. In a horizontally integrated organization, the patient is usually stationary, and the organizational units tend to have duplicate or complementary, rather than shared, medical services. They are more likely to share administrative services.

The relationship between two hospitals can begin with horizontal integration, with both belonging to a shared service program, and then change to a vertical arrangement as referral patterns begin to be affected by the new relationship and a two-way flow of patients begins. Obviously, sharing administrative services is much simpler than sharing medical services.

Management Implications

Within a single hospital, activities are usually highly specialized, interdependent, and interrelated, so when multiple hospitals are linked with other types of health service units, the implications for management processes are significant.

The Impact of Scale on Leadership

The administrator of a 400-bed specialty or tertiary hospital operates with clearly defined levels of authority and responsibility, and a staff that includes associate and assistant administrators. He or she is responsible for providing leadership and direction. By sheer physical proximity to a single institution's problems, the administrator can help associates and assistants mature and cope with change. The management processes can be nurtured daily.

If the scene shifts and this chief executive officer provides management for units geographically separated by distance or organizational characteristics (i.e., group practice), additional challenges will be encountered. The chief executive officer has to cope with the frustrations of directing from a distance, without the luxury of day-to-day contact. This can be frustrating for the traditionally trained executive who is used to operating with team members close at hand. In establishing linkages, the chief executive officer will undertake a greater risk when selecting a manager for an outlying unit. The new manager will have to accept centralized management while still providing on-the-spot decision making. Achieving economy of scale through centralized control will be a greater challenge since more autonomy is being given to the remote unit manager.

As the number of units increases, pressure grows to create a corporate structure. Controls must be established through the development of specialized management and reporting services. Financial officers, purchasing agents, and other staff specialists will be making visits to the remote units. However, centralized management services must be sensitive enough to the process to avoid detracting from the autonomy of the local unit manager, which would create vulnerability and have an adverse effect on managerial growth. (One of the most difficult issues to quantify is the "value added" associated with centralized corporate oversight and direction. A number of large multi-institutional systems must constantly justify this overhead to their constituent parties.)

It is essential that leaders work to discover the appropriate balance between centralized and autonomous management. Economy of scale may actually be less important over the long run than the need to initiate strong, effective local management by administrators who can function without a high degree of over-the-shoulder advice and control from a central office. In terms of the internal operation, the attempt to remove barriers between departments in a single institution frequently is countered by the managers' understandable need to maintain control of the decision-making process within their own departments. These problems increase in complex linked structures with more vested interests.

Management Philosophy

The leader can help to bring about a solution to this management dichotomy by ensuring that the organization has an articulated managerial philosophy. The simple principles outlined below may reduce the level of friction and frustration in the multiple unit operation.

1. Linked institutions should operate with a single set of written objectives relating to patient care and administration. These objectives should be reviewed annually and serve as visible symbols of common purpose.

2. Administrators of the organization must be able to identify with broader group missions, and CEOs should keep this need in mind when hiring new members of the management team.

3. Department heads within individual units must be discouraged from playing one unit off another. Usually there are a number of shared services found in these organizations, and managers should be encouraged to operate with their mutual dependence in mind. A hospital, for example, may furnish engineering services to an adjoining group practice. A request from the group practice administration for engineering services should receive the same service priority as one from a hospital department, even though the engineers are hospital based. This is a very important aspect of management philosophy, and it must be supported by those in an integrated operation.

4. If possible, administrators should be rotated from time to time from one unit to another, and transfer preferences should be given to those who most closely identify with central mission statements. The movement of managers in this way will reinforce the importance of understanding the overall program. All managers should be charged with responsibility for maintaining systemwide discipline for organizational policies and practices, and should also command respect for company culture.

5. Adequate overlap should be developed in board, medical staff, and administrative assignments, and top executives should be vested with more than one responsibility; for example, an administrator of an adjacent group practice could function as a board member of the hospital. Chief executive officers, in particular, must place a high priority on maintaining this type of organizational surveillance.

Allocating Management Time

Today, hospitals and other health care institutions still appear to be undermanaged. Too many administrators seem unwilling to bite the bullet to allocate more dollars for enhancing management processes. Under these circumstances, multi-institutional arrangements must be approached with great caution. It is much easier to "close the deal" on a service relationship with a second institution than to produce an end result that will be a building block for future arrangements instead of being the weight that sinks the ship.

The issue of centralization versus decentralization of management must be addressed when expanding a multiunit program. Should a corporate headquarters be developed and staffed with individuals who function as system specialty managers, or should management consist of a local unit manager who is linked with an existing associate or assistant administrator in the larger urban center? One advantage of developing the core corporate staff is the creation of a structure with precise assignments and priorities. The drawback is that those who operate as members of this core may be confused (and legitimately so) by having to deal with a wider spectrum of detail than those who have limited internal operating responsibilities. On the other hand, creating a separate core staff can detract from the unit administrator's opportunities to participate fully in developing internal systems and managing the total process. As a result, the unit manager may have a harder time developing enthusiasm for the total management process.

Although the more traditional approach in multi-institutional organizations is to develop a core staff of specialists to manage the process, there are alternatives that can work very effectively. One variation is found in an urban-rural network system where the rural hospital administrator is matched with one of the administrative officers in the larger urban hospital. Within this system, each of the four or five local unit administrators has an in-house contact. Shared core staff people can be mobilized more rapidly because of the vested interest that the urban hospital staff administrator develops in the remote or related unit.

The Leader's Role and Responsibilities

Cooperation

Success in building relationships with other institutions and health facilities depends on support and endorsement from the top. The chief executive officer does not develop a program by dispatching an assistant administrator into the field to make an arrangement. The appearance of organizational arrogance must be avoided, and chief executive officers of larger institutions must recognize that they may be out of touch with the complexities of operating smaller hospitals or health care units. The executives of larger hospitals have backup and expertise available, but the administrator of a smaller hospital operates as a generalist, without any overlap in staff responsibilities. It is very important for the relationship between two units to be enriched by active participation and involvement between the chief executive officers, regardless of the size of the units involved.

In an urban-rural linkage, it is critically important that each executive refrain from imposing his or her organization's values on new colleagues in the alternate setting. A 16-bed coronary care unit in a large hospital does not operate with the same set of problems found in a 2-bed combined surgical special care and coronary care unit in a 25-bed hospital in rural America. Relationships between institutions prosper when institutions and their leaders recognize their role in responding to needs rather than creating them. The urban center is not necessarily the best place to make all decisions on the needs of smaller units.

Use of Power

The application and use of power varies with circumstances and style, and one potential danger associated with larger, more complex structures is that the individual executives are in a position to acquire and use power to their own advantage. Organizations grow as a result of strong leadership, and the chief executive officer needs to acquire a power base. On occasion, though, some executives lose sight of the mission of the organization and begin to build an unhealthy personal power base.

Some people think that the aura associated with a powerful individual leader, as manifested in extravagant expenditures such as exotic suites and private airplanes, stimulates or symbolizes organizational growth and prosperity. But if not used with caution, these manifestations of power can become destructive. More than one organization has fallen on hard times because of the failure of the executive or the institution to recognize the pitfalls of power and the need for balance. Humility is a valuable commodity and a particularly useful characteristic for executives in multi-institutional arrangements.

Building the Team

The success of linked organizations depends on how well the organization and its leaders are able to develop the management team. The way the management team works together is usually reflective of individual management styles. The leader should help managers recognize the types of decisions that can be made at lower levels in the organization, and the team should try to avoid investing too much decision-making power in a few individuals at the top. An egocentric chief executive officer who stresses a top-heavy vertical structure can easily deprive the organization of its full potential.

Separate units in a multiunit system should be encouraged to exchange information horizontally and should operate as task-oriented teams. Members of such teams should even try to forget that they are associated more with one unit than with another. If this philosophy is successfully applied from the top down, the process will encourage strong management teams.

Staff Burn-Out

The pressures on executives in linked structures are severe. Fail-safe systems should be created to prevent depleting the energy of these individuals. The cumulative effect of pressure can eat away at executives' abilities and endurance. Although individuals ultimately must be responsible for identifying their own limits, the system has a responsibility to avoid overstressing any individual for a prolonged period of time. Second-level executives, medical staff colleagues, and board members should be mindful of the fact that natural leaders often operate with a disproportionate amount of missionary zeal and will often expend more physical and mental energy than is healthy or even desirable.

The chief executive officer has a responsibility to protect the organization and should select a number of staff who are willing and capable of sharing the demanding work load. Too much reliance on a single individual is an invitation to disaster. The field has lost some superb executives because they failed to recognize that energy is not a limitless commodity. The career paths of some of these individuals have been like the flight of a meteor!

Adapting Styles to Cope with Growth

Matching administrative style to institutional needs in a rapidly changing system is an important challenge in establishing organizational linkages. The CEO of an urban center that is acquiring management interests in nursing homes, group practices, or home health care agencies needs to address this issue carefully since he or she may have to select an administrator to manage the new unit. It is important to look at individuals' previous experience and personality when determining whether or not they are suited for the job. An individual who performs well as an assistant administrator in a large unit may be a poor director of a smaller self-contained unit.

There are also significant differences in the kinds of management styles needed to function effectively in different settings. For example, nursing home administration demands a different approach than managing an acute hospital facility. Since relatively little "career crossover" takes place in the administration of different types of health care institutions, the pool of administrators trained in two or three different types of management is limited. Differences in administrative backgrounds will add a dimension to the linked organization that will have to be addressed by the chief executive officer when coping with growth.

The leader can help by making a conscious effort to nurture newcomers. If the organization's goal is to successfully develop a multiunit program, the CEO must remember the importance of continuity and contact with individual administrators. Young administrators need role models. Making sure that they maintain contact with chief operating executives will help in retaining good young executives and will provide the chief executive with a means of selecting future leaders.

Planning

Long-range planning is an overworked phrase, and few will quibble with the desirability of creating a ten-year plan. Most multi-institutional system executives know that growth frequently results from the ability of someone in the organization to recognize and take advantage of immediate and unanticipated opportunities. So while long-range planning is an essential part of establishing an overall direction and setting guideposts along the trail, high priority must be placed on developing short-term flexibility. Managers should be encouraged to recognize valuable immediate opportunities. Management support systems should respect and reward individuals who are able to leap to a proper conclusion without being encumbered with facts. Some of the finer achievements in organizational growth result from contingencies rather than long-range plans.

Five Factors in Success

Although many health care systems undertake the process of organizational linkage simply for self-preservation, a well-integrated multiunit organization should be able to achieve the goal of providing better patient care at lower costs. Appropriately linked systems are said to deliver better care because units use an approach to patient services that is based on a broader, less fragmented perspective. Many linked organizations specialize in administrative or management services because they are easier to share than medical services. But executives in these organizations should also turn their attention to establishing shared medical systems. Better coordination of care beyond the hospital walls can mean the difference between a patient's rapid recovery and a slower, more prolonged recovery. It is important to pursue anything that can be done to move the patient gently through various stages of care without the gaps in care that seem too often to occur once the patient leaves the hospital. Linking medical resources narrows these gaps.

Why does one linked system prosper while another one fails? The answer may lie in part in these five factors:

1. Successful ventures occur in organizational frameworks characterized by financial growth, stability, and innovative leadership.

2. Successful ventures are found in organizations that are outwardly driven by virtue of the need to develop a broader service market for long-range survival.

3. Successful ventures are backed by management teams consisting of individuals who possess enthusiasm and missionary zeal and who operate synergistically.

4. Successful ventures need sufficient management reserves to cope with brush fires and still manage the future.

5. Successful ventures are found where leaders are perceptive and open to new trends. Although in the past emphasis has been placed primarily on multihospital organizations, the future calls for expanding linkages with different types of health care institutions, including group practices, nursing homes, and home care services.

Conclusion

There is a certain magic in the success of linked organizations, but that does not make the process easy. Executives in multi-institutional units should always reflect carefully on the management implications associated with expansion. Success depends on the ability to change management styles, to accept new commitments, and to recognize the possibility of personal and organizational vulnerability.

11

CONFRONTING QUALITY AND COSTS: AN ACTION PLAN FOR EXECUTIVES AND PHYSICIANS

Case in Point

Dr. Louis Nielson, the CEO of Graystone Medical Center, was perplexed. At a recent Rotary Club meeting, a panel of health care purchasers (those buying health care for their employees) had stressed their concern about rising health care costs. Their solution was to promote competition between providers to drive down the costs of health care.

Dr. Nielson was particularly disturbed by the fact that no one expressed concern about the quality of care. If costs were reduced without any attempt to measure the impact of cost reductions on quality, patient care might suffer. Why was everyone missing this point? Dr. Nielson reflected at length and then appointed a special task force to figure out how quality, in addition to costs, could be factored into the health care equation.

What the task force discovered was that Graystone, along with most other providers of health care, was unable to really prove that they were providing health care that matched the purchaser's definition of quality. Health care providers traditionally focused on clinical outcomes (i.e., whether or not the patient survived and healed without complications). But what employers really wanted to know was whether or not the patient (employee) recovered in a timely fashion, whether or not he or she was satisfied with the care received, and whether or not he or she was able to return to work quickly. In other words, was the health care received valued highly by all parties? This represented a much broader definition of quality than reflected in outcomes alone.

As a result of their studies, Graystone Medical Center began to invest heavily in developing systems that measured these and other "value" factors. Subsequently, they were able to convince purchasers of care that Graystone not only delivered high-quality care that was cost-effective but also that the medical center focused on the value of the care to the patient.

Like the search for the Holy Grail, the health care leader's quest for quality is never ending. Administrators in health care face many obstacles, are subject to unpredictable events, and need stamina, courage, and humor to stay the course as they continue to try to balance the issues in the debate over cost and quality.

The worst side of competition has surfaced in price discounting for an illusionary market share. Tantalizing new technology is increasingly unaffordable. Traditional insurance companies are facing serious financial drains and have raised premiums significantly. Without sufficient resources for developing a better data base, we continue to make decisions based on a fragmented system that is distrusted by many but still used to justify new regulations. And this brings continued increases in the amount of litigation. (thus the speculation that law schools are now graduating two attorneys for every physician completing medical school). The cumulative effect of all of this, of course, is that health services executives and physicians are facing increasing numbers of confused, angry, and distrustful patients.

One of the most eloquent descriptions of today's health care environment was delivered by Paul Ellwood in the 1988 Shattuck lecture. Ellwood said:

> The intricate machinery of our health care system can no longer grasp the threads of experience. The mischief that began long before the health care crisis of the 1970s is progressively disabling the vast machinery of medicine. Too often, payers, physicians, and health care executives do not share common insights into the life of the patient. We acknowledge that our common interest is the patient, but we represent that interest from such divergent, even conflicting, viewpoints that everyone loses perspective. As a result, the health care system has become an organism guided by misguided choices; it is unstable, confused, and desperately in need of a central nervous system that can help it cope with the complexities of modern medicine. The problem is our inability to measure and understand the effect of the choices of patients, payers, and physicians on the patient's aspirations for a better quality of life. The result is that we have uninformed patients, skeptical payers, frustrated physicians, and besieged health care executives.[1]

Is lower quality the price you pay for cost containment? Does increasing quality necessarily mean driving up costs? The bottom line is that the cost versus quality debate, which reached its peak in the 1980s, has left us with more questions than answers in the 1990s. Health care leaders will be called upon increasingly over the next decade to work toward resolution of the debate. We know now that the first step is understanding and agreeing on what we mean by quality in health care. The second step is giving physicians, who have borne the responsibility and pressure of demands for quality, the support they need to continue their excellent work.

The Role of Physicians

There is a perception in the field that we cannot really define what we mean by quality in medical care because the diagnostic and treatment atmosphere varies so substantially from one setting (or patient) to another. But even though quality may be difficult to define, we all know good care when we see it. Most of us recognize the following factors as representative of high-quality medical care, regardless of the particular situation or setting[2]:

- Good outcome—as measured by mortality and morbidity data (standardized and compared with others)
- Efficient use of resources—as evidenced both by practice pattern effectiveness and by the physician's recognition and response to the over- and underutilization of resources (as well as responsiveness by the professional to the use of demonstrated effective protocol)
- Appropriateness of care—based on when and how the service is rendered (whether, for example, it is appropriate to perform an asymptomatic hernia repair on a patient with terminal cancer)
- Patient satisfaction—an essential factor because a satisfied patient responds better to diagnostic or treatment suggestions (and becomes more involved in healing processes) than does the uninformed, uninvolved, dissatisfied patient
- Evidence of a program to further improve quality processes—by devoting adequate resources (both finances and personal energy) to the continual assessment and further improvement of the trajectory toward a predictable outcome in diagnosis and treatment

Most of these characteristics are directly tied to the performance of physicians, and for that reason, physicians are shouldering the burden of maintaining quality of care in the health care setting. At the same time, because physicians are in a vital position with regard to health care spending, we also hold them accountable for escalating costs.

Physicians under Fire

Nowhere is the constant tension between cost and quality more evident than in the work and daily responsibilities of physicians. The volatility of the environment with regard to costs makes it very difficult to see clearly on issues of quality, and physicians are in an extraordinarily difficult position with respect to defending quality in patient care delivery. Because physicians control 60 to 70 percent of health care expenditures, they have become the obvious target for society's frustration over the astounding increase in U.S. expenditures on health care. Yet most physicians go into medicine because they are interested in patient services, so they are angry that patients and society are beginning to "take them apart" and challenge their traditional professional prerogatives.

Meanwhile, in many areas of the country there are too many physicians in selected specialties, so physicians themselves are being forced into competition. They go deeply into debt to complete medical school and residency training. They make family sacrifices in order to achieve their goals. Yet as a group, physicians have a relatively short professional career. Practicing physicians deal constantly with unpredictable events that can put them in a battle siege mentality until they eventually burn out. They rank high in statistics relating to divorce, addictive problems, and suicide—a clear indication of the level of stress they endure.

Now data banks that display practice pattern variations have contributed to putting physicians on the defensive. Studies of physician practice patterns raise many questions about the kinds of decisions doctors make. Why, for example, do operative rates for caesarean sections vary substantially from one community to another and from one insurance plan to another? Why do physicians in the same specialty on the same hospital medical staff take different approaches to the diagnosis and treatment of similar patients? In some cases, varying practices may simply reflect the physician's training, since training practices certainly vary in different hospital settings. In other cases, though, practices vary because individual physicians have standardized their approach to a particular kind of case without necessarily studying what would work best in other related cases. Once physicians participate in well-structured data base studies that identify the correlation between outcome and practice patterns, these old habits usually begin to change. Quality is enhanced and costs are usually reduced. Yet initially such programs are threatening. Physicians who know that their practice pattern variations are being scrutinized often feel that their professional medical prerogatives are being compromised.

Future Implications

Obviously, physicians are in an uncomfortable position. We expect them to guard standards for quality and at the same time keep costs under control. If we continue on our current course, the way that health systems function in the future will depend largely on four issues:

First, will physicians be able to practice more effectively? Can they operate with fewer resources but provide the same outcome?

Second, how will physicians accept the inevitable changes in compensation and payment systems? Will these changes lead to conflicts between physicians that will jeopardize their ability to work collaboratively to ensure the delivery of cost-effective, high-quality medicine?

Third, will healthy patient-physician relationships survive in the face of the public's growing frustration about costs? Will these frustrations translate into lesser quality?

Finally, are physicians capable of providing the leadership required to deal with quality issues in the face of retrenchment, or will quality issues be left to third parties (government, insurance companies, and so on)?

How Can Leaders Help?

What is management's role with respect to quality? As some physicians might be inclined to ask, what business do administrators have in becoming involved in the issue of the quality of medical practice? The leadership objective is to develop a corporate culture that includes quality as a key component. The leader is responsible for influencing physicians, nurses, and others to become involved in a total commitment to caring about quality. Obviously, this means that administrators must be proactive and influential rather than passive and acquiescent. In addition, they must rely on wholehearted support from physicians since quality enhancement programs are never successfully developed by administrators alone.

Executives have an obligation to be sensitive to the patient-physician relationship and to understand as nonphysicians that they have obvious limitations with regard to understanding the practice of medicine. But they should not sell themselves short just because they are not trained in medicine, nor should they be apologetic about asserting what they know best. The way an administrator handles the complexities of problem solving in administration is similar to the way a physician approaches the review of multiple patient complaints to arrive at a diagnosis.

Leaders who are interested in being proactive on the issue of quality within the practice setting should recognize the limits of their expertise but not be overawed by physician credentials. An amazing number of decisions on quality are based on common sense. Because quality of care issues are so closely linked with the appropriate consumption of resources and the costs involved, the leader's expertise and input are invaluable.

When examining quality in medical practice, leaders should also emphasize objective data. Physicians are more likely to respond to objective information used to demonstrate a point than they are to subjective conclusions made about their work. One way to go about collecting objective data is by creating and monitoring a patient complaint response system. Make sure that the feedback loop is complete and that the system is not viewed as an administrative system for surveillance. The system should involve physician leaders, nursing leaders, and others.

Quality-of-care programs will be most effective if they appeal to the innate desire of professionals to do good work, so leaders should be consistent in their emphasis on maintaining quality assessment systems. Executives must exemplify consistently high professional and personal standards and promote these standards throughout the organizational setting. Quality should be a topic of concern at all levels and to all audiences in the organization.

To increase the organization's awareness of the importance of quality, leaders should take the time to define quality in their own terms and then involve others in working toward an organizational definition. Quality should be viewed as an attainable goal, and leaders should look for opportunities to identify specific actions or events that have contributed to improving the quality of care provided by the organization. Since good quality is viewed by some as an elusive characteristic, it helps to define it in the context of day-to-day operations. For example, establishing a formal and effective patient complaint review system makes an obvious contribution to improving the quality of patient services. In addition, a program to make services available to more patients supports quality in the sense that the increased volume is necessary to maintain clinical expertise. Leaders should make the relevance of these measures known to staff at all levels in the organization.

When encountering problems with the quality of physicians' work, administrators should use peer pressure—physician to physician—to help work out solutions. Physician leaders should be involved in bringing about changes in physician practices (and the same goes for nurses and nursing practices). Avoid bypassing the medical governance structure so that the existing structure does not become an inadequate mechanism for coping with the tough issues of quality.

Leaders should be careful not to act on poor or inadequate information. When you are dealing with issues of quality of care, guesses are not good enough. Do the job thoroughly. If you launch a quality enhancement program without carefully analyzing the processes and without using multidisciplinary teams to come up with the right questions to ask, the program may bog down.

The quest for quality requires leaders who can recognize system weaknesses and who are willing to do something about them, even in the face of some risk. The process is time-consuming and there are no shortcuts. However, leaders who truly recognize the importance of improving the quality of health care are usually willing to invest the resources and energy needed to develop quality enhancement programs. They are the leaders who will contribute the most to changing the health care system in the years ahead.

Establishing Priorities for the Next Decade

Administrators, board members, and others who are engaged in the quest for quality must work closely with physicians to alleviate some of the pressure that physicians bear. The health care system of the future will need to be transformed if it is to be freed of the complexities that have made it a hostile environment in the past. Health care leaders are in the best position to influence the decision making that will bring about the necessary transformation. Among the reforms needed are the following:

1. The health care system should consist of organizations and individuals who subscribe to an integrated cooperative approach to health care (rather than a competitive model).

2. A system must be established to allow providers to operate under a predictable cost structure.

3. Physicians, executives, nurses, and others will need to function as partners in a unified effort to enhance quality.

4. Those who purchase care must emphasize not only cost but also quality and outcome when making purchase decisions.

5. There must be concurrence among providers, patients, and payers as to what really constitutes good quality.

Exploring Outcomes Management

Executives who want to take steps toward improving quality must first become believers in the concept of outcomes management, which means that they must be willing to participate actively in developing and using data systems that pinpoint and recognize effectiveness and efficiency in the practice of medicine and in the consumption of health care resources. Simply correcting the financing mechanisms or investing more money in the system will not work. A fundamental change in approach is needed.

Leaders will have to invest human and financial resources in the effort to develop a feedback loop with respect to improving both hospital- and physician-based methodologies for medical practice. Although many have criticized the release of hospital-specific mortality data by the Health Care Financing Administration (HCFA), the release of the data has had the interesting effect of forcing providers to pay more attention to the power of centralized data. The amount of data held by insurance companies and the federal government is extraordinary and ultimately will force change whether providers like it or not.

Consumer guides to physician-specific mortality and morbidity rates will follow. Providers have a choice of either waiting until this happens or being proactive and willing to contribute to the development of data bases and the use of such data to adjust internal practice patterns. Leaders would be wise not only to encourage their organizations to participate in this trend but also to make it easier for physicians to participate in developing the data bases as well. One of the keys to getting physicians to accept this concept is to make certain that the processes are physician driven. We can begin by identifying and supporting physician leaders who will take the time to lead the program and who will embark on the process by fostering an attitude of self-improvement through education, rather than pursuing data banks as a means of humiliating poor performers.

In spite of the growing propensity for organizational retrenchment and the developing siege mentality among physicians, leaders must focus their energy on building effective response teams. Building teams means focusing on what is important: the patient. The team leader's role in this process is to lead by example and to keep the team focused on the important issues. One way to do this is to work constantly to build a service mentality—to strive at every opportunity to demonstrate that the patient does come first—and to look for ways to recognize those members of the team who promote that attitude.

Although organizational stability is essential as the means by which hospitals or group practices and other providers obtain resources to support quality measurement and control systems, financial stability and prosperity cannot be the leader's sole objective. Leaders must function in a businesslike fashion to survive, but if they are going to ensure excellent care they will have to define quality in a way that consumers and purchasers of care will accept, and to measure quality in a tangible and consistent way that goes beyond the bottom line.

An Action Plan for Quality Improvement

The quest for quality is built upon a thorough understanding of the critical relationship between quality and cost. Reducing the consumption of resources does not necessarily result in a reduction in quality. In fact, in many instances, a reduction in the use of resources actually improves quality. One of the foremost experts on quality, Edwards Deming, has taken this concept a step further to suggest that if you improve quality, costs will go down. The concept of decreasing costs by increasing quality is a strategy worth considering carefully as we brave the stormy weather ahead. An action plan to effectively improve quality and control costs involves seven steps:

1. Enhance the visibility and participation of physician leaders because they must be ready and willing to confront the issues of quality and costs before the rest of the medical community will follow. One way to accomplish this is by providing financial assistance to enable physician leaders to visit other organizations that have ongoing quality improvement programs.

2. Elicit physicians' help in identifying practice pattern inefficiencies. (This step is difficult but absolutely essential.)

3. Whatever the individual physician learns about his or her own practice efficiencies should be recast in the light of a broader educational effort to share information with specialty subgroupings.

4. To manage resources appropriately, physicians should understand the financial impact of their decisions. Physicians must be convinced that they are treating both the patient and the patient's pocketbook.

5. The identification of test procedures and other services that are underutilized is the step most often overlooked. Underutilized tests obviously also contribute to poor outcomes (mammography is a classic example). Physicians and executives who are able to recognize underutilization probably know how to obtain and analyze practice pattern study information in depth.

6. An effort should be made to upgrade the understanding, evaluation, and selection of severity-of-illness systems. These systems must measure outcome, efficiency in the use of resources, and the appropriateness of care. At this point, severity indices in hospitals are more highly developed than in the ambulatory setting. However, since so much health care in the future will be rendered in the ambulatory setting, a reliable severity-of-illness system for ambulatory care must be found. (There are several systems available, but at this time there is no universal acceptance of any of the models.)

7. Finally, leaders should accelerate the development of mechanisms to measure the cost-effectiveness of the physician's practice. The issue is cost, not price. Although we see our mission as developing high-quality care that can be provided at an acceptable price, pricing care at an appropriate level suggests that the true costs of producing services are understood. Costs must be emphasized in discussions of quality. Needless to say, it is impossible to deliver services below cost for very long before quality is affected.

Conclusion

The ultimate test of health services leadership is the leader's ability to persuade others to rally around causes and missions that honor and respect human values. As health care executives are increasingly pressured by external and internal events, they must not abdicate the responsibility to serve with physicians and other professionals as guardians of quality.

Continuous quality improvement systems have to be directed toward making it easier for physicians and other providers to diagnose and prescribe, and for patients to collaborate actively in the healing process. Although it will take great energy, personal courage, and total commitment, executive leaders must work with physician leaders and others as advocates for the quality of that interchange.

Notes

1. P. M. Ellwood, "Special Report: Shattuck Lecture—Outcomes Management: A Technology of Patient Experience," *New England Journal of Medicine* 318, no. 23 (1988): 1550.
2. L. F. Fenster, "The Case for a Change in Medical Practice at VMMC to Ensure Survivability into the 21st Century," Report of the Physician Practice Patterns Task Force, Virginia Mason Medical Center, Seattle, August 1988.

12

THE ANGUISH OF DOWNSIZING

Case in Point

Mountain View Hospital Medical Center seemed to be on solid ground. It was located in a growing suburban community and was surrounded by a number of physician office buildings. The census was averaging around 75 percent. The closest neighboring hospital was 15 miles away. The medical center's board consisted of prominent community leaders. The administrative team had experienced little turnover and the administrator's credibility was high.

The community was shocked one morning to read newspaper headlines indicating that layoffs of hospital employees were imminent. According to one hospital administrator, the newspaper reported, the hospital needed to trim its operating budget by 10 percent. The article also revealed that the hospital had lost money the previous year in spite of the high level of activity. The reporter implied that mismanagement was the cause of the trouble. The administrator countered by stating that such cutbacks were routine in the health industry and that the responsibility rested with payers, particularly the state and federal governments, because they were compensating the hospital at less than actual costs.

In fact, what occurred at Mountain View was the direct result of three key problems. The first was that in an era of prosperity (high census) the executive staff had implemented a grand strategy for expansion. Building projects had been ongoing for six years, and too much capital was consumed too quickly. The interest and principal payments exceeded predicted levels. The second problem was that the operation was at risk due to discounting arrangements made with preferred provider organizations and other payers in order to capture market share. These concession rates proved to be very expensive because the arrangements did not produce the volume of patients expected. The third problem was that high levels of accounts receivable had affected the center's cash flow and forced the organization to use up its credit line.

Any one of these problems alone would have been severe. The combination of all three seriously shook the confidence level of board members and the medical staff, and ultimately led to the termination of the chief executive officer and other members of the management team. The lessons—avoid overexpanding (control capital), monitor discounts (concessions) closely, and keep an eye on current operations (receivables)—were all learned the hard way.

We will all be affected by whatever lies ahead in the health services industry. Some say that it will not get worse, but most of us think it is more likely that it will. We have already seen the turnover rate for hospital CEOs climb from 16.9 percent in 1980–81 to 24.2 percent in 1986–87.[1] More recently, the rate has hovered in the 18–20 percent range. Turnover among executives in group practice settings appears to be running at approximately the same rate.

As external events begin to take their toll on individual organizations, administrators are spending increasingly more time on resolving internal operating problems. And as problems occur internally they tend to reduce their external monitoring. It is important to remember, though, that if the world is going sour and you are not continually tracking new external developments, it may only be a matter of time before your organization is hit by another jolt from the outside. A second, or third, or fourth jolt, when unexpected, could be devastating to the organization.

Proposals for restructuring the entire health system are surfacing in Congress. Many of these proposals call for action to require mandatory assignment for Medicare payments to physicians, which would prevent physicians from billing patients for the difference between the federal fees and usual and customary charges. Physician fee schedules will soon be controlled through the implementation of the resource-based relative value scale (RBRVS), which establishes for the first time a national cost-based physician payment structure by specialty. Capital costs could be capped through establishment of limited capital pools for which hospitals would have to compete. Volume of procedures would be controlled by creating volume norms, which if exceeded by the provider would force payment adjustments in succeeding years.

Reducing or restructuring the organization is one of the most difficult things a leader will ever have to do. If and when the time comes that this is necessary, however, the leader needs to be prepared. Assuming the environment does get worse and your organization faces an urgent need to turn the operation around, what should you expect? What can you do to ease the transition when the organization faces cutbacks and restructuring? How can you create the right climate for a turnaround and get the organization back on its feet?

Early Warning Signs

Leaders need an early warning system to alert them if their boat is leaking or if they are about to sail into a hurricane. There are a number of specific indications that an organization is in trouble, and leaders should always watch for and guard against these warning signs.

Cycle versus Trend

Month-to-month income variations based on a changing number of revenue days per month, or expense cycles that fluctuate, are cyclical. But when you use your computer graphics program to plot the last three years of revenue and expenses, making adjustments for price increases, and you see a line aiming in the wrong direction, it is not a cycle anymore—it is a trend.

Executives sometimes confuse a cycle with a trend, making serious problems worse by trying to fix them with short-range solutions. For example, relying on price increases rather than expense reductions to reach an acceptable bottom line is a short-term solution. No longer can health care organizations be managed by simply manipulating the revenue structure.[2] Leaders must adjust the orientation of the management team in recognition of the fact that short-term financial fixes will not work and that organizational restructuring may be necessary. Positions may have to be eliminated, and employees will need to be cross-trained. Management teams must be energized to permanently adjust basic cost structures.

Deviations from Budget

Leaders should be attentive to deviations from budget plans. Traditionally, we monitor comparisons between budget and actual relative to revenue and expenses. But do we spend enough time forecasting changes in patient mix and fluctuations in net revenue that result from volatile discounts from third party payers? It is a revelation to see what happens to discount rates if you increase prices but fail to watch the payer mix.

Sloppy Business Decisions

Some of the greatest mistakes of the last decade have resulted from too much reliance on pure historical data and a failure to incorporate predictions about market trends into the formula for the future. For example, some physician groups have excess office space in new buildings because when planning the project they simply ran their historical volume lines into the future. They did not take into account the projected shifts that would occur when employers moved groups of employees from one managed health care plan to another.

Several years ago, Boeing Aircraft in Seattle suddenly moved thousands of employees and their families from a private insurance carrier to the local Blue Shield Preferred Provider Plan. This had more than a modest impact on physicians and hospitals that were not members of Blue Shield's preferred provider organization. Providers (hospitals and physicians) who were not members of the preferred provider organization experienced firsthand the health benefit purchasing power of the employer, and they developed a new appreciation for the need to monitor insurance arrangements that might limit access to their organizations.

Failing Commitments

Executives need to track ongoing commitments to monitor the cumulative effect of their decisions. For example, the overall effect will be significant if you add a new physician and support staff in one specialty, purchase several pieces of expensive high-tech x-ray equipment, and contract for a building addition. Carelessness in tracking the cumulative financial effect of adding expenses and debts that will affect the organization in the second, third, fourth, and fifth years, particularly when combined with the loss of volume, can create significant problems. The leader must focus on the big picture and learn to ask the right questions about the strategic scene to avoid getting lost in detail.

Excessive Borrowing

If cash reserves shrink and it becomes necessary to borrow to meet monthly expenses, the organization is in serious trouble. Some borrowing can be expected when organizations are expanding, but your cash flow should not be so tight that you find that you are constantly borrowing to meet monthly expenses. If you are borrowing to meet current expenses, an immediate sequence of corrective actions should be taken to curtail expenses. Long-range forecasts should be examined very closely. Planning should be initiated to build reserves, and the board should be carefully briefed so surprises are minimized.

Too Many Distractions

Another indication of trouble is when an administrator begins to encounter a series of unrelated crises that distract his or her attention from routine business. As the pace quickens, administrators can become consumed by specific projects or problems, and in the process they may lose track of basic operational issues. For example, failure to keep an eye on accounts receivable can precipitate a genuine cash crisis. More than one capable executive has lost the game by ignoring the gradual buildup of receivables, and the seasoned executive should know that even in a state of crisis it is important to keep tabs on routine budgetary issues.

As a side note, although bankers seem to be quite willing to lend money to organizations that are doing well, they also know how to tighten the thumb screws very quickly if they do not like what they see. Particularly in recent years, bankers sometimes have had very short memories.

Threatened Credibility

We can probably all recall colleagues who suddenly found themselves unemployed. Some of them may have been persistent in their belief that they were in control of the situation and could turn it around in time. Their inability to accurately and effectively relay critical information may have compromised their credibility and undermined their relationship with their board.

Boards have the capacity to absorb only so much bad news before they react with a decision to "shoot the messenger," and this places the administrator in a rather tenuous position. Taking all the bad news to the board means you must be ready to take the heat. But it is also very dangerous to sanitize bad news, protecting board members from the severity of the situation in the hope that the situation will turn around. If it does not turn around, you must face a group of extraordinarily agitated individuals who are ready to take action against you. The manipulation of facts to distort the news, to make the situation look either better or worse than it is, can easily lead to the destruction of leadership credibility.

The antidote is total disclosure. Without alarming the board, the leader needs to paint a realistic picture of the organization's state of affairs. It should be possible for the leader to give the board all the facts and figures without necessarily suggesting that the organization (or its leadership) is out of control. Rather than panicking or giving an overly gloomy forecast or withholding information, the leader can inform the board members of the current status of the organization's programs and give them the actual figures, but at the same time focus the board's attention on the steps that are being taken to address specific goals and issues. Making sure the board knows that you are in control will help to preserve your credibility.

The Challenge to Leaders

Coming to Grips: The Leader's Reaction

When an organization is faced with a financial downturn, leaders tend to respond in a somewhat predictable pattern. First, they often try to deny the problem, believing initially that it is "only a blip," a "self-correcting trend," and that all they have to do is wait it out. In the denial stage, the administrator searches for reasons why the problem is temporary and not very serious. All kinds of excuses surface: "We miscalculated concessions but it has now been corrected," or "Our receivables are up temporarily but we can get them down in another 60 days," or even "You remember that snow storm we had last February—it affected volume more than we thought." The executive will use any excuse to deny the need for action.

The second stage is delay. All sorts of short-range strategies and explanations are employed: "All we need to do is work a little harder and the problem will disappear," or "We need to study alternative solutions more thoroughly to be sure." Suddenly it takes three quarters to prove a trend, and the leader suggests, "Let's wait until the end of the year to see how it looks." The decision-making time line begins to stretch and stretch and stretch.

And then things don't get better. In fact, they get worse. The third stage—depression—begins. Everyone starts to get a little anxious and the inevitable question is raised: "Why didn't we act earlier?" The organization's perpetual pessimists, who always predict catastrophic events, begin to clamor: "We're in a tailspin—we'll never recover now."

Depression is like a virus, and it affects employees, managers, and physicians alike. Some begin to think that it is time to bail out. Unfortunately, if panic sets in, it is often the best people who leave first. A feeling pervades the organization that nobody is in charge. Quality and the capacity of leadership are challenged. Board members may begin to propose unrealistic solutions, which if adopted precipitously, create a series of fire storms that add to the pressure.

In some organizations, supervisors, employees, and physicians will use the crisis as an opportunity to play games, to consolidate their positions, and most interestingly, to dissociate themselves from those leaders who are associated or identified with the downturn. Their mood can be conveyed in a single idea: Distance yourself from the problem if at all possible.

And then suddenly the organization's true leaders dig in and resolve to correct the problem. As decisions are made, attitudes begin to change. Stories of problems experienced by other organizations begin to spread throughout the clinic. Leaders sometimes even look outside for some bad news because it helps physicians and others understand that some of the internal problems are caused by external environmental conditions. Soon a more optimistic attitude is revealed in conversations: "We've experienced rough times before. Why is this so different?" "Look at how the department managers are responding to this crisis. We have the capacity to turn this thing around." The healing process is under way, morale is improving, and the leaders are beginning to move down the playing field toward the goal line.

The Role of the Board

If anxiety about the organization's stability is increasing, there is usually an inclination on the part of board members to become more involved and more informed, which tends to translate into more frequent meetings. The problem with increasing the frequency of meetings, however, is that each meeting needs to be properly staffed, and if you increase the frequency of meetings, you begin to run the risk of making decisions on the spur of the moment without adequate staff input and research. Decisions that are inappropriate will end up needing to be reversed, so you might as well take your time. Resist the inclination to meet too often, particularly if the meetings require a lot of preparation.

There are a number of ways to cope with increasing pressure from the board, but the most basic strategy is to ensure that board members are totally informed of what will be done to rectify the situation and to involve them in the decision-making process from beginning to end. Failure to keep the board informed destroys the trust that is essential to organizational and personal survival.

The executive faces a more difficult task if board members seek, either individually or in small groups, to implement their own solutions to a problem. It is important in this case to bring the board together in the process of making decisions by organizing projects, such as fact-finding initiatives or the preparation of environmental position papers, that will bring home the point that the whole field—not just one organization—is in turmoil. These activities should be designed to get to the root of the problem while at the same time building the credibility needed for organizational renewal.

The Role of Managers

Administrators who have been through tough times know that they cannot always predict how supervisors will respond to a crisis. Some managers are flattened by crisis and find it difficult to cope. Others rise to the occasion, and although they may not enjoy what is going on, they are challenged by the circumstances and may actually flourish in the crisis situation. They suffer the pain and anguish of downsizing, but nevertheless they get the job done. And because they have confidence in themselves and their organizations, they can live with what they have had to do because they truly believe in the greater cause. These supervisors are an immensely valuable asset; they need to be nurtured and supported.

Leaders can support supervisors by anticipating crises whenever possible and preparing the management staff for needed change. Off-site educational opportunities in which supervisors can learn from managers who have faced similar problems in other organizations help to give support to the supervisory role. Personal networking should be encouraged so that when problems occur, external and internal resources are available to help supervisors cope. Finally, managers and supervisors who respond well during times of crisis should be rewarded for their behavior. Personal recognition from leaders, in addition to appropriately timed financial recognition, will help supervisors know that they are valued and will give them motivation to continue their excellent performance.

Building a Turnaround Atmosphere

When undergoing downsizing, an organization needs a strong administration with solid leadership and values. Leaders who have emphasized the following priorities will find that all of the steps in the process of getting the organization back on its feet—including downsizing—will run more smoothly.

Strong organizational values. An organization that has a history and culture of doing right by people will be better equipped in troubled times. When times are rough, some organizations become shortsighted in dealing with people who might be let go, as well as with the people who remain. If the organizational culture is based on human values, as reflected in its service to patients, this attitude will prevail through the time it takes to turn the organization around. Retrenchment issues will be dealt with more sensitively, and the organization as a whole will recover with more speed.

A credible executive staff. Goodwill increases when leaders accomplish good results for the organization and the people in it. The deposits you make in your goodwill bank today will go far toward guiding you and the organization through hard times in the future. If your goodwill bank is depleted because you have not invested sufficient time and energy in building organizational assets, you will find that you have little reserve in times of turmoil. This message holds true for the entire executive team, who should constantly monitor their leadership credibility to ensure that they are in good standing both within the organization and in the larger community.

The team approach. An administrator who is a solo performer—who believes, for example, that physicians have little business in administration—and who goes about attempting to build and protect administrative turf, is doomed to experience a short tenure. The administrators who survive volatile times are those who understand the importance of involving physicians in decision making. It is a symbiotic (and synergistic) relationship between physician leaders and executive administrators that provides solutions to tough problems. And the same goes for the rest of the health care team.

Difficult Decisions

You have sized up the problem, and you have elected to work a strategy of increasing volume, with a focus on reducing expenses. This means convincing a lot of people that they are going to have to work harder with less support. Department managers have combed through their budgets at least three or four times. Those with flabby budgets and those who have secreted away a few surpluses have been identified and asked to make the necessary cuts. The moment of truth has arrived. Unfilled positions have already been frozen, so that's not the solution. The time has come to choose which individual employees within the organization will have to be terminated.

This is where the anxiety peaks. Do you lay off by seniority or by level of competence? If you are heavily unionized, you may not have a choice. The impact of laying off senior employees should not be underestimated, however, since it begins to tear at the fabric of the organization. A number of important factors will have to be weighed as you consider these difficult decisions.

Where and How Much to Cut

Recognize on the front end that the problem is probably more severe than you think it is, and make your personnel cuts deeper than you believe is necessary. The reason for this is that the planning will not all fall into place easily. Some executives tend to underestimate the magnitude of the problem, and if they have to go back to the managers for a second or third cut, they lose a tremendous amount of credibility.

There will always seem to be some compelling reason why an individual whose position has been eliminated should be kept on by the organization for a period of transition. Except in a very rare instance, resist the temptation to drag things out—transitional periods usually do not work well. Individuals who have had their position taken from them are shocked and angry. Rarely can they tolerate working in a different capacity for the organization that has let them go.

Be cautious about thinning out your administrative staff. As anxiety increases in the organization, executives will be pressured to respond. Lack of administrative support can itself contribute to the problem, since it is the resource most needed to cope with the tension and turmoil associated with layoffs. Think of the big picture: Will curtailing the organization's capacity to respond to new threats work to the organization's disadvantage?

When reductions in expenses are taking place and people are losing their jobs, wages are usually frozen and benefits are cut. Be careful about reducing benefits. Some long-term morale problems will occur if employees believe that everything is being taken away from them.

Yet another thing to think about is the impact of downsizing on the physicians. Executives typically cut back in non–patient care areas first, protecting quality by leaving the direct support staff of the physician groups intact—and this makes sense. In reality, though, what you may have to do to meet your target is cut back on medical records, medical secretaries, and other support personnel that really do affect the physician. The point is that it is essential to include physicians in the process on the front end. Do not keep them in the dark about what is coming or try to cover up the impact that the layoffs will have on their practice.

Separation Packages/Support Services

Do not try to get by with a cheap separation package. When you are letting people go, you want those who leave to feel that the organization has been fair and cares for them, and you also want those who are remaining to feel that the organization was fair to those who left.

Track the employees who leave to make sure that they are well placed. Make certain that department heads and others are supportive of those who have lost their jobs and that they are willing to go the extra mile on references and job assistance. In spite of the magnitude of the crisis at home, you cannot afford to forget those who have been terminated. Extra attention is essential not only for the sake of those who leave but for the sanity of the employees who remain.

Planning and Communicating in Crisis Situations

Plan the events involved in the downsizing process carefully. If outplacement services are available, work out specific arrangements ahead of time. Rehearse with your supervisors how information is going to be presented to the individual losing his or her job. Once a decision has been made and everything is in place, make the cuts cleanly and with compassion. If those who are leaving feel that they have a support system in place and are being well taken care of in terms of severance pay and outplacement services, everyone will sleep a little better at night, although it may take some time.

Frankly, it is very important to move individuals out quickly, but try not to move people out of the building so quickly that they do not understand the commitment of the organization on their behalf. Support services are absolutely essential. When one well-known insurance company went through organizational restructuring, they fired several of their top executives without prior notice, and on telling them that they were through, the chief executive officer, in an astonishing case of bad judgment, had the senior officers escorted off the premises by security guards, refusing to let them return to their offices to say farewell to their secretaries and collect their personal belongings. This type of action is totally uncalled for and will haunt the entire organization for years to come. The rift between senior executives and other employees in this instance is so severe that the wounds may never completely heal.

The humane and appropriate approach is carefully thought through in advance of the necessary separation. Separating packages should be as liberal as possible, and the announcement should be well timed and crafted to be as straightforward as possible. Outplacement counselors should be present to meet immediately with the affected personnel. Shortcuts in the process will be quickly interpreted by the "survivors" as callous and insensitive. The leader is responsible both for seeing that the proper action takes place and for handling the situation in a fashion that does not further impede the organization's recovery.

Communication with Physicians

During a crisis, it is easy for physicians to get left out of the communication loop. Executives often overlook the importance of communicating with physicians when they are focusing on the rest of the employee force. As a result, physicians may be in the embarassing position of hearing important news from their office assistants or hospital technicians. Leaders should be attentive to the way they communicate at all times, making sure that physicians always receive information firsthand so that communication does not break down during crises.

There are a number of ways to improve communication with physicians. For example, the administration at Virginia Mason Medical Center in Seattle created a series of special topic mini-seminars for its medical staff. Attendance at the seminars was limited to 25 physicians to allow for discussion. The seminars addressed several topics in depth; among them were updated financial information, strategic planning, prepaid plan activity, retirement benefits, cost containment, and other items of special interest to the physician. Some seminars were well attended, others were not, but we were able to condense the information and disseminate it to all interested parties, making sure that the physician board of directors were the first to receive the briefing material on each of the seminars so they would be in a better position to communicate with their peers on the staff.

Another process that works well, if thoughtfully done, is to prepare special newsletters designed specifically for physicians. Although physicians might appreciate the organization's general employee newsletter, there is a lot of information that would be of particular interest to physicians (recognition of physicians for special accomplishments, information on net revenue, new program developments, and so forth).

Of course, all of these activities consume staff time. They are not easy to plan, especially if you have thinned down your administrative staff. When you engage in these new programs, you must be committed to expending sufficient energy and resources to make the programs succeed. Starting a program and stopping it in midstep does not speak well for your follow-through and leadership credibility.

Communicating Bad News

An organization in the midst of a retrenching program faces a lot of major questions simultaneously, and executives have a tendency to try to make one decision at a time and disseminate the news slowly. The problem with this approach is that you keep reminding the organization of how bad things are. It is probably better to clump bad news together and send it all at once.

It is also wise to monitor the means and content of the material that others are sending out in your organization. This is particularly true in the large organization where memos come out from department chiefs, various administrators, and supervisors. Although they may all be well-intentioned, these memos do not necessarily carry the same message. Uncoordinated messages, no matter how well-intentioned, will only add to the organizational disarray.

Dealing with Rumors

When you are downsizing, rumors are rampant. Look for ways to confront and deal with them before they become destructive. One way to handle them is to establish a hot-line telephone number for employees to call to get their questions answered promptly. You can measure the mood of the institution by the number of calls received. Open employee forums are also good for keeping messages intact. Whatever the method, creating alternative opportunities for employees to communicate is important.

Leadership and Morale

Administrators and managers need to be highly visible during crisis times and should not shirk their responsibility to explain to employees why they are being separated. It is important that individuals know that the layoffs have nothing to do with their performance but are the result of unfortunate economics.

When you have gone through downsizing, there are many employees who are affected. Imagine, for example, an administrative section where several secretaries have been released. Imagine yourself walking down the corridor and seeing empty desks and quiet phones. Think of what that sight would do to your remaining employees. Desks should be removed and new configurations and work assignments developed quickly so that empty spots do not serve as constant reminders of the problem.

There is always a lot of gallows humor that accompanies an organizational crisis. Some of this is healthy but some is not. Laying people off is not something to be taken lightly. Sometimes the most innocent expression of humor in front of a group of employees can cause a serious backlash, particularly if the humor is considered inappropriate, untimely, or insensitive. Humor in the face of the anguish of others is always inappropriate, so choose your words carefully or they may come home to haunt you.

As layoffs begin, make sure that management staff members have been thoroughly briefed and that they understand the reason for the layoffs. Executives should be able to explain the matter honestly and directly, and should give thought in advance to how to articulate their explanation consistently.

Timing is important in working to improve the morale of the organization. Instinctively, executives will try to pull everyone together in group meetings and talk through the problem. But sometimes this is just too painful. Sometimes a little time is needed to allow some emotional healing. Two years after our organization went through some downsizing and an individual was moved to a lower position, the manager of that individual's department was still unable to refer to the incident without getting choked up. We were scheduled to have a management retreat during the downsizing process, but we elected to cancel it because the morale of the supervisory group was so bruised that it would not have been a useful exercise.

The point here is that some healing time is required. About six months after the event, the first management-wide social event was held, and it was a great success. It was organized by a team led by an executive who had previously appeared to be aloof at such occasions. Skits were organized to help bury the past and prepare for the future, which helped bring about the healing process that was so badly needed by supervisors, managers, administrators, and other members of the management team. We had turned an important corner and would be in a better position to facilitate healing throughout the rest of the organization.

Conclusion

The health services environment is already worse in some parts of the nation than in others. Preparation for the tough times ahead must include the refining of external environmental surveillance systems that will ensure that you and your organization are not caught off guard.

It is essential to work harder than ever before to build the strongest possible management teams. Know the strengths and weaknesses of your supervisors, and surround yourself with capable people. Keep an eye on the mission and culture of the organization. Too much attention to isolated parts of the operation (for example, stressing only financial performance) will inevitably affect the health and vitality of the organization and will detract from its reason for being.

Finally, never underestimate the amount of energy that will be required to turn an organization around once it is in trouble. If you think you can work yourself out of the problem simply by producing, and without addressing expense reductions, you may be in for a long, cold winter. And if you think expense reductions are a one-time event, you will probably find out that you are wrong; from here on out, reductions will be the routine, not the exception.

When confronted with the challenges of the next decade, the survivors among us will somehow pick their way through the mine field, choose the right course of action, and demonstrate optimism even in the midst of anguish. This optimistic outlook for the future is crucial; it provides a source of stability for the organization. Leaders do not lose hope. They display courage, consistency, compassion, and competency, minute by minute, hour by hour, and day by day.

Notes

1. P. Weil, A. Wilhouse, III, and M. Caver, "Hospital CEO Turnover: National Trends and Variations (1981–1987)," *Healthcare Executive* 4, no 1 (1989): 42–45.
2. J. Goldsmith, "A Radical Prescription for Hospitals," *Harvard Business Review* 89, no. 3 (1989): 104–11.

PART IV

VISION: LOOKING BACK
AND THINKING AHEAD

13

TAKING STOCK OF YOUR CAREER

Case in Point

In July of 1991, I celebrated 36 years at Virginia Mason Medical Center. One of my mentors in the early years was John Dare, who was also my predecessor as senior administrator. He used to kid me by saying that I seemed incapable of finding another job. The truth was, though, that I never really wanted to find another job.

It wasn't that I didn't have offers. In fact I explored several, perhaps more as a means of reassuring myself that I was doing well by my family than because of any real need to move on. One of the opportunities was particularly memorable: it not only offered professional challenges but also a salary that was 40 percent more than what I was earning at the time.

So why didn't I move? Very simply, because I liked what I was doing. I was fortunate enough to be working for a great organization that valued quality. The medical staff excelled. The board recognized the difference between policy and practice. There were opportunities for advancement, and most fundamentally, no two days were alike. It was exciting and I liked the people. They made me feel that I was helping to improve the organization. Yes, there were problems and frustrations and systems failures. But the organization was supported by a corporate culture that demanded the best of the individual.

In the 70 years since Virginia Mason began there have been three senior administrators, and I am the third. I am one of the lucky few who found professional opportunities that matched my personal and professional goals.

But many of the physicians and other administrators have spent their whole careers there too. They seem to know that they too can make a difference. And that is about all any of us can hope for.

No one in an organization is indispensible. An institution's structure survives long after its founders and subsequent generations of physicians, executives, and employees have disappeared. Organizational momentum carries the institution forward, and in the process, there are many different hands at the helm. Even the most competent health care executives sometimes wonder how to survive in this volatile environment. In fact, any administrator who does not think about survival must either be playing a very safe game without taking any obvious risks (although playing it safe is a risk in itself), or existing in an oblivious state, without any "surveillance systems" to indicate what is going on outside the executive office. Executives who look realistically at their environment are bound to be dealing with a lot of pressure. They need to know how to recognize symptoms of personal stress and, more importantly, how to cope with them.

Now is a good time for many of us in health care to take stock of what we have accomplished in our careers, and to establish a plan that will maximize our leadership effectiveness in the taxing years ahead. Are we the outgoing, confident executives we seem to each other to be—or is each of us just getting by without any "program" for handling the stress in our daily work life? Designing a personal strategy for survival allows us to cope with today's pressure so that our "springs don't snap," and so that we can live to enjoy the fruits of our labors. This chapter focuses on identifying and coping with stress in the profession, the importance of reexamining career and personal goals, and when to look ahead toward retirement and the future of the organization under new leadership.

Stress and the Health Care Leader

We all know individuals who have been stressed in the worst possible way, who have encountered great personal tragedy and disaster, and yet have matured in spirit. Most of us also know someone who cannot handle stress at all. Successful health care executives must be willing to accept and be committed to understanding the stress inherent in their profession. The individual who has really learned to cope with stress—who knows both how to reduce it and how to live with it—will usually stand out in a crowd. They seem not only to anticipate stressful times but to be aware when symptoms of stress start to take on a life of their own.

Hospital or clinic executives who are winding the spring too tight display very specific symptoms. They tend to

- Put in long hours on the job
- Leave no time for recreation
- Accumulate lots of unused vacation time
- Keep a hand in everything that is going on
- Get bogged down in detail
- Try to please everyone
- Find it difficult to complete projects on time
- Find it difficult to make decisions
- Lose their temper more, particularly at home
- Have few, if any, close friends because they are too busy to cultivate friendships
- Find it difficult to communicate with their spouse, children, and other family members
- Seem tired much of the time and do not really look forward to the future
- Seem uneasy, uncertain, and even a little panicky on occasion

Stress and Leadership Style

These days the buzzwords in discussions of appropriate leadership styles— "participatory management," "team management," and similar terms—reflect an interactive relationship between management and staff. We are advised that we should be close and sensitive to those we manage. However, this style of leadership lends itself to a particular dilemma for those of us who have built our careers as straightforward and assertive managers. How can someone who is used to being the authority and giving directives suddenly become sensitive and participative? And how should we respond to the pressure to change?

If you know you are a top-notch executive and you follow solid management practices, objectives, and goals, then your management style is probably right for you. Resist changing in a way that will make you into something you are not. You have to march to the tune and beat of your own drummer, and old-fashioned directness is not a sin. It is not necessary that you conform, only that you recognize differences in leadership style. If you are weak in one area, you should surround yourself with staff who have strengths in that area. If you find it difficult to display sensitivity, make sure you have a manager who is comfortable expressing concern for individual employees and their involvement on the staff. Be realistic, and do not tilt windmills unless windmills are your specialty. Life is too short to spend time fighting both your environment and yourself.

Stress and the Mature Executive

Executives are said to go through three stages in their professional growth with regard to their attitudes and managerial style. Young executives fret about the inability of those around them to grasp their new ideas. They are more likely to play the odds and take risks in decision making. They are on the move and their confidence appears unlimited, although they are sometimes naive and misdirected. Mid-career executives have been bloodied but are still unbowed. They have developed a seemingly effortless decision-making style. They convey a sense of confidence that is valued amidst today's turmoil. Late-career executives have acquired wisdom and experience, which anoints them as elder statesmen. Less inclined to make hasty decisions, they have a rifle shot instinct for what is right and wrong.

In *The Great Jackass Fallacy*, Harry Levinson reports on a survey performed by Lee Stockford of the California Institute of Technology.[1] In Stockford's survey of eleven hundred men, about five out of six men in professional managerial positions said they had experienced a period of significant frustration when they were in their mid-thirties, and the survey noted that one in six said they had never fully recovered. If the study had included women managers, it probably would have revealed similar (or more) frustration among women in their thirties, whose career choices may be compounded by decisions regarding having and caring for children.

Middle age is the critical age when executives come face to face with reality and find that reality does not always measure up to their dreams. Age itself, of course, does not have to be a barrier. Sophocles lived to be more than 90 and wrote *Oedipus Rex* at 75. Benjamin Franklin invented bifocals at age 78. More recently, Benjamin Beaggar, Professor of Plant Physiology at the University of Wisconsin, was required to retire at the age of 70, but he then proceeded to join the research staff of Lederle Laboratories and invent a new antibiotic.

Admittedly, these are exceptions. Perhaps it is more typical for middle-aged executives to slowly become frustrated until finally they accept that their actual performance and position may never measure up to their earlier ambitions. This too is an important lesson since failure to recognize that real life does not always measure up to one's expectations will eventually cause even the best executives to become bitter.

Early in their careers, young executives can afford to build a "castle in the sky" without having to face the realization that they might not reach their goal. But when executives reach their forties and fifties, they have to begin to adjust their goals more realistically. Rather than worrying about whether the crown will look good on them as they sit upon the throne, executives begin to worry about whether they can even swim the moat in order to reach the castle's portcullis.

To look at it from a slightly different angle, the young executive can develop all kinds of innovative ideas and can carry them off with a flash of enthusiasm. But older executives have the advantage of being able to sort out these ideas more easily. Middle-aged executives' mystique, which helps contribute to their success, is based on the ability to draw on years of experience when looking for solutions and making decisions. When older executives find the hounds snapping at their heels, they can rest assured that they are more likely to cross the finish line ahead of their younger competitors, simply because they know where to find it.

Survival Tools

How do you go about improving your capacity to survive? Mature health care executives should concentrate on developing new attitudes and sharpening old skills that will help them live and cope with the pressures that abound in the health care arena. It is important to consider what your strengths as a leader have been in the past, what they are at present, and whether or not they will be sufficient as we make our way through the trying 1990s. Do you need new skills, more training, new ideas? Will your tried-and-true approaches sustain you under pressure? The suggestions below are intended to address the evolving concerns of the mature health care executive, although they certainly apply to executives at any stage in their career.

Setting priorities and making decisions. When you are under pressure, try to maintain a sense of routine in daily activity. What really begins to push one over the edge is not the number of decisions that have to be made but the type of decision. Decisions that carry a high risk, such as proposing new services or significant policy changes affecting physicians and patients, take a greater toll on the executive than will decisions affecting more routine activities. You can avoid becoming overloaded by setting priorities on decision making. This does not mean putting off making difficult decisions, it only means that you should strive to make decisions in a sensible order. Do not put off decisions that need to be made immediately, and do not waste time deliberating over decisions of little consequence. When you find it is becoming more difficult to make decisions, you should sit down and assess whether you are overloaded.

Addressing stress and life issues. It is important to identify issues that add stress to your life as well as activities you enjoy that help relieve stress, and then try to maintain a balanced perspective and lifestyle. Your performance at work is dependent upon how complete you are as a person, so you need to evaluate your physical and mental health, your involvement with your family, and any other personal factors that play a critical role in your general well-being.

Staying in good physical shape helps people of any age to function better mentally and to relieve physical and emotional stress. A reservoir of strength and vigor helps the individual cope with the pressure of the daily demands of the job. Although this may be one of the first things we let slide when the pressure is on, we all know that physical and mental health are equally important in a well-rounded lifestyle. We also know, but must continue to remind ourselves, of the importance of diet and exercise in reducing stress and maintaining personal health.

For some, middle age is a shattering experience that affects home life as well as professional life. Couples who once shared common interests with their children may find that their children are gone and their romance is a bit shaky. It is important to recognize this as a normal process and to work with family members when confronting some of these midlife frustrations. It is difficult for a family to prosper if they are always given short shrift.

Even seasoned executives may need to be reminded that their families need and deserve special attention. Many of us who got caught up in developing our careers at an early age may have had to readjust to regain our balance at home. Ambition is useful. Success in a career is important. But it can be a lonely life for those who never learn to find the right balance between family and career. Knowing your own values will help to keep your career in the right perspective.

Managing time. It is not so much the early morning meeting, or the responsibility of working a major project through the board, or the rebellious teenager at home that creates the overload. Most of us can handle these isolated incidents. It is the cumulative effect that creates the problem. If we could resist the temptation to fill every minute with activity, we might find ourselves with some spare thinking time. How many meetings do you attend that could just as well be attended by someone else? Unfortunately, because of our puritan work ethic, many of us feel guilty if we are not busy all of the time, and this cumulative busy-ness is, in itself, stressful.

To manage your time most effectively, you need to learn to tap your personal rhythm, to know when your mental chemistry is up to the task of creative thinking. Everyone has up days and down days, but to be creative you have to ride the waves. Some of the most productive days follow dog days. You need to develop your own devices for keeping a balance that allows you to be productive without being pressured. Try making a list each week of immediate and long-range tasks. List both tough tasks and easier ones and scratch them off as they are completed. This helps to keep you moving ahead in the right direction. Cultivating such devices will be your salvation when things begin to pile up.

Keeping current. Executives become obsolete more subtly than do machines. Obsolete administrators may not even be aware of their deficiency and may rely on self-protective defense mechanisms to keep them from facing their own flaws. Frequently, it is the environment that changes, and the executive who has failed to monitor the changes is at risk. Keeping current by monitoring the literature, networking with colleagues, and being aware of your strengths and weaknesses is of utmost importance.

One of the best ways to stay in the know is by making an active commitment to teaching, since conveying knowledge requires discipline and the ability to stay one step ahead of your students. Regardless of whether your students are undergraduates, graduate students, or your peers, the process of teaching requires new information and ideas.

Maintaining networking skills also helps the health care leader stay informed. By keeping track of people, visiting with colleagues, and attending continuing education programs, executives are able both to become more educated and to exchange information with their peers. If you are not already doing this, you should be. Consider yourself a receiver and transmitter of information. Bring the news home. Work diligently to develop new professional relationships in other parts of the region and nation. Visit other institutions. All of this requires a commitment of energy and effort, but it is worth it for the depth it will bring to your career.

Networking should not be limited to relationships with peers (at the same level of experience and responsibility) or superiors. A key benefit of networking is the contact it allows with those who are younger and perhaps less experienced. Younger colleagues may be closer to a newer information base and may challenge your thoughts and ideas. In doing so, they are making a valuable contribution to your success by helping to keep you current.

When to Quit

In every career there are key landmarks. Decisions are not without costs, and when you decide to leave an organization you do not always know that you are making the best decision. If the building is burning down around you, and you stumble across a bucket of tar and a box of feathers in the board president's office, perhaps the decision has been made for you. It is more likely, though, that well in advance of tar and feathers, you will be able to pinpoint landmarks along your career path and assess what it is you are really accomplishing and, more significantly, whether or not it is worthwhile.

Although a considerable number of individuals in their forties and fifties change career paths entirely, little has been written about the process of deciding to move on to something else. When have you given enough? When have you given too much? Here are four questions to consider if you are thinking about moving out of your organization and on to another, or out of your profession entirely:

1. When you go to work in the morning, do you look forward to work, or is it a continual drag? Do you view your work as a challenge or as an anchor?

2. Are you so comfortable in your organization that you are able to predict what each of the board members or physicians is thinking? Are you so comfortable that you use these predictions to make decisions? If so, you are probably becoming complacent about decision making, and that is a risky position. Your alleged extrasensory perception will soon be resented by your colleagues, staff physicians, and board members who are not provided with the courtesy of full involvement in your decision making. If the challenge is gone, and you are at the point where you are beginning to act on assumptions rather than on reasoned facts, your decision as to whether or not it is time to quit may soon be taken out of your hands.

3. What is the status of your goodwill bank? You need a surplus of goodwill to get things done. To maintain personal credibility, integrity, and confidence, leaders should avoid letting their goodwill bank go empty. Every time you make a good decision, solve a problem, or contribute toward the organization's goals, someone somewhere will make a deposit on your behalf. However, if you make poor decisions, or even if they are correct but unpopular, people will be very willing to make a withdrawal. If your goodwill bank is wiped out, you will be forced to operate with a deficit.

If you have drawn too much from your account, you may have to consider whether it is time to quit and move on. You can usually rebuild your goodwill bank if you still have enthusiasm for your job. But if your level of enthusiasm and vitality also happens to be in a deficit mode, you had better think seriously about where you are heading.

4. Are your principles intact or are they being compromised? This is a very important question. If you feel your usefulness to the organization is minimized because you cannot agree with what it is you are doing every day, you should think seriously about your future. If they are good at what they do, health care executives cannot survive very long when their principles—their philosophy and attitude toward problem solving, for example—are being compromised. If you have consistently tried to enforce personnel policies, assuring employees that policies will be applied fairly to all, you will be dismayed to find instances where managers are violating procedures and getting away with it. But when you start to overlook these deviations, your personal code of behavior is eroding, which spells trouble as well as loss of peace of mind—and, ultimately, the potential loss of your position.

Considering Retirement

At some point each of us will decide that, rather than moving on to another organization or taking on new responsibilities where we are, it is time to give up some of our responsibilities to others and to focus more on our personal affairs. Retirement means different things to different individuals. Regardless of how you view it, you will be happiest if your preparations are made well in advance.

To some, retirement comes easily. They are the executives who make their preparations early, taking advantage of advice and information from financial consultants, human resources specialists, and their own health care providers. They look forward to pursuing interests and hobbies left undeveloped during their careers, and they enjoy being in control of their schedules without constantly being on call for meetings and professional commitments. Their financial resources have been harbored carefully, and their vested retirement funds were carefully rolled over and protected each time they changed positions. These executives have taken the time to work with their spouse at preparing to have the high-charging executive suddenly spending lots of time at home.

For others, though, the scenario is quite different. Particularly if they have not thought ahead and done some planning, they may encounter a whole host of personal difficulties when adjusting to their separation from their work. Perhaps foremost are the potential financial implications of retiring. Nine out of ten health care executives probably ignore the need for careful financial planning and may even end up running short when they retire. It is easy for executives to move from one position to another, using up retirement funds to make down payments on houses and to take care of other family needs. People who work in health services might be particularly apt to overlook personal financial requirements as they pursue their mission to serve patients and the organization, but they will be in for a rude awakening when suddenly faced with a severely restricted budget.

Beyond the financial adjustment, the loss of identity can be agonizing for the professional who moves out of a position of authority and into retirement. Suddenly, your advice is of less importance. Friends stop calling, not because they have any less interest in you as a person but because you are no longer in the communication loop. (How many times have you called and visited with a retired colleague?) To make matters worse, it may be necessary to build new friendships with people with different interests, since many friendships developed over the years are with other health professionals. Building new relationships, according to some senior citizens' publications, is supposed to be easy and productive. But if your interests are very specialized, new friendships cannot be developed without a lot of hard work. In addition, as old friends pass away or confront disease, the reminder of mortality may weigh heavily on the new retiree, who suddenly has plenty of time to ponder what lies ahead.

If the retired executive has not developed hobbies or interests (other than professional ones), retirement will bring the need to find a way to fill time. Interests and hobbies that were allowed to wither because of the press of the job may no longer be of interest. (It is more difficult to climb a mountain peak at age 65 than at age 32.) Although travel is often held up as one of the antidotes to the loss and separation from a regular job, the executive may identify travel with work, not pleasure. There have already been too many airports and hotels, and travel may not hold the glamour it once did.

A whole new set of hazardous conditions may surface at home when the new retiree is suddenly spending lots of time around the house. This has to be one of the final tests of a strong relationship. The retiree might try to help by taking on extra tasks but might end up disrupting routines in the process. Authoritative attitudes from the job may be hard to curtail, creating new kinds of turf issues when applied at home. If both husband and wife are retired and are now in close proximity day in and day out, dependency relationships may change. If neither spouse is bringing in an income, the couple's standard of living might need to be adjusted, and this can lead to additional opportunities for conflict.

The list of possible problems is seemingly endless. The purpose of this particular recitation is to emphasize that retirement should not be taken lightly. When asked how they are enjoying retirement, new retirees often answer enthusiastically. "It's great! You should try it!" they say. Be careful about accepting that response at face value. Just as when fully employed, the retired executive typically seeks to achieve but may find it difficult to admit that retirement is not all that easy. Each individual has to work out a personal and workable solution. Trial and error will demonstrate which tactics are most helpful, but there is likely to be some pain along the way.

Some Helpful Hints for Survival

There are some things that can be done to ease into retirement with all of its benefits, rewards, and problems. The first is to really plan ahead. Never wait until the last moment to start getting ready. Financial planning for retirement starts with one's first job, and active retirement planning should be initiated no later than age 60. (Many experts will suggest that retirement planning should begin even earlier than age 60, but this is difficult to do.)

The planning should focus first on what you want to do when you leave your current position. This means more than just figuring out how to fill those freed-up days. If, as is true with many leaders, you plan to continue some type of work and professional involvement, begin by identifying activities that you *like* to do and consider building your plans around them.

Leaders often think of going into consulting as a good way to spend their time in retirement. Consulting is hard work that demands time and energy. To respond to your client's needs, you must stay professionally up to date. If consulting is among your identified interests, examine all the opportunities available to you and make sure you understand what is involved. A false start can be dangerous in retirement because you do not have the support systems afforded by an established organization.

One approach to organizing your time is to develop a strategy that includes two or even three professional activities such as community service, teaching at a local college on a part-time basis (teaching is also very demanding of time and energy), or involvement on business or corporate boards. Develop some short-term relationships to try out the activity, but be careful not to overprogram yourself. Learning to deal with some down time is essential.

Look for situations that offer the following conditions:

- Control over your time and calendar (teaching, for example, requires a commitment of time for a specific quarter or semester, but regular office hours may not be required year-round)
- Flexibility in work setting and environment
- Access to a central office that is equipped with a fax machine, copy machine, and computer (a home office should include a modem)
- Adequate and predictable income, so that financial fluctuations are minimized and retirement principal is not consumed
- Intellectual stimulus and control over externally generated professional pressure
- Professional satisfaction and support
- Year-to-year flexibility
- Enough free time for recreation and leisure
- Freedom to enjoy and be responsive to important personal relationships

At the same time, reexamine your leisure time likes and dislikes. Do not feel obliged to participate in typical leisure activities just because others do. If you are a golfer, fine—but many of us are not. (My predecessor, John Dare, loved golf, but he also became an accomplished painter during retirement.)

It is especially important to keep your spouse involved in all of your retirement planning. You will need advice from your partner. Share your concerns fully and there will be fewer surprises later. Keep in mind the possible impact of your move from office to home. (I remember asking my 90-year-old uncle, who had been retired for many years, about his secret to successful retirement. He said it was very simple. Always get up at a reasonably early hour and clear out of the house between 10 A.M. and 3 P.M. In his case, he and several of his retired friends employed a secretary and shared several small offices downtown, so they had a place to "get their mail" and "watch their investments.") If you like working at home, set up a special room and keep it equipped, but do not expect that your spouse will enjoy acting as your secretary! Make use of all the helpful new technology: a fax machine and a modem on your personal computer can help keep you in touch—that is, assuming you wish to keep in touch.

Other clues to preparing for retirement include (1) anticipating the shock of the change, (2) checking your health status and controlling bad habits, (3) accepting the necessity of going through retirement parties (they are essential for those you are leaving behind), and (4) above all, understanding that there is no set formula for ensuring a successful transition.

It has to be personally tailored and tested—and then continually modified along the road.

Every individual takes a different approach to the prospect of retiring. Some do it by launching a second career, while others elect to really change their lifestyle. Some leaders will be as compulsive in retirement as they are in their careers. If you are one of those very fortunate ones who can approach retirement full of enthusiasm, and if you never want to dabble in health administration again, then by all means kick up your heels, ignore much of this advice, and design your program accordingly. Whatever you choose to do, as a leader in the health services field, you have earned every minute of it.

A Word about Succession Planning

The sense of achievement that goes along with success often contributes to a sense of responsibility for the process of selecting a successor. As they prepare to leave the organization, some health care executives might start seeing themselves as indispensible and, as a result, might even try to clone themselves by picking and promoting a successor who possesses leadership traits like their own. To those who slip into this mode of thinking, I would offer this word of caution: Be careful about taking an overly active role in picking your successor. Organizations that are fortunate enough to have been led by a successful executive have usually had that executive around for a long time. When a senior executive retires, the organization needs to make the most of the opportunity to look over its leadership needs and create the team best suited for the future.

But how can an executive who has carefully and deliberately developed and nurtured a strong management team just take a back seat and let nature take its course, particularly when the board of directors may not know all of the strengths and weaknesses of internal candidates? Senior executives who have been devoted to team building understand that one of their primary responsibilities is to see that team members are continually profiled. If the CEO has claimed the limelight and overshadowed the accomplishments of others, the organization will suffer during the transition. If the executive has truly been a successful leader—in terms of profiling members of the management team—board members should be knowledgeable about team capabilities, and the retiring executive should be able to back off a bit from the process.

Although each person's situation is different, all retiring executives should spend time thinking through the transition and helping to prepare the organization for the process. Listed below are some suggestions to keep in mind as you think about your organization's future:

1. Set your retirement date far enough in advance that the organization has time to consider the implications of the change. (A year is a good time frame.)

2. Although you have set the date well in the future, be prepared to move it up if succession planning moves along well. Once a successor has been identified, the incumbent needs to be prepared to move out of the way.

3. Turn over the reins as soon as is reasonable. Try to avoid the tendency to hold on until the last day; this simply puts decision making on hold and temporarily freezes the organization's progress.

4. Do not leave in a rush. Certain ceremonial events (retirement dinners and so on) need to occur before you go. These events are important both for those who are left behind and for the leader who is leaving.

5. Be calm, cool, and reflective as the process unfolds, and think things through from the organization's perspective (rather than just a personal viewpoint).

6. Complete most of your long-range personal planning well before you announce your retirement so that you are not diverted by having to make significant personal decisions when you need to be working out those essential organizational processes associated with a changing of the guard.

7. Once the organization has settled on a successor, support the decision all the way. It is very destructive to take a neutral position after a choice has been made by the board. Be helpful and enthusiastic about the organization's future.

Not all departures are voluntary, and succession planning is a whole different matter if you are leaving the organization under less than pleasant circumstances. What posture should a health care executive take if the decision to find a new leader is made elsewhere in the organization? Even leaders who are being forced to retire or otherwise leave the organization have a responsibility to rise above the situation and depart with as much grace as can be mustered. Those left behind will be particularly troubled by not knowing what the future holds for them. Particularly in times of organizational turmoil, a new leader will bring in a new team, and this can have a devastating effect on the old team. With this in mind, the outgoing leader should try to take a philosophical approach to the situation rather than expressing anger and creating further distress within the organization.

In spite of the difficult circumstances faced by the outgoing executive, nothing is gained by leaving behind a trail of accusations and bad feelings.

The ability to rise above the circumstances and make an orderly and dignified departure is a sign of greatness in any individual. In these situations, it is wise to disengage promptly because the organization will be paralyzed during the interim between the old and the new.

Organizations cope best with transitional issues if the leader who is leaving, whether the departure is voluntary or involuntarily, understands the big picture and—hard as it may be—keeps his or her emotions under control. The wise executive instinctively knows when to quietly intercede in the selection process and when to leave it alone. The ultimate objective, after all, is to leave the organization better off than when you joined it. This requires both wisdom and the ability to separate personal goals from those of the organization. One's goal should always be to leave with grace and a personal sense of having done it right.

Conclusion

If you sit around feeling sorry for yourself and make no effort to understand what is going on around you, then you can expect to encounter some rough sledding in the years ahead. You can increase your creativity and control by learning how to live with stress rather than resisting or succumbing to it. We all encounter stress, but those who really make it—not just as professional executives but in all aspects of life—are those who have really learned to cope, and to live comfortably with themselves.

How do we learn to flourish in an arena filled with confrontation and pressure? The key is to start by developing a personal strategy for survival based on what you want out of your career and your life, and to cultivate your mental flexibility. Surviving means being involved, making a personal plan, and modifying it to meet new and special circumstances. Success in life does not happen accidentally. It is a process of training and development that never ceases.

Note

1. H. Levinson, *The Great Jackass Fallacy* (Cambridge, MA: Harvard University Press, 1973).

14

TOUGHING IT OUT: LEADERSHIP
PRIORITIES FOR THE YEAR 2000

Case in Point

It is the year 1994, and federal legislation mandating a single payer system has just been passed. The insurance industry fought the legislation, but to no avail. Frankly, as the CEO of Southern Cross Medical Center, a tertiary hospital of 500 beds, you are more than a little relieved just to know what lies ahead. Through the past several years, the system has been gradually falling apart. The access situation has worsened to the point of becoming intolerable. Underinsured patients are literally unable to find critical medical services because reimbursement systems have reduced payments to hospitals, physicians, and other providers.

You have already leaned down expenses as far as possible without threatening quality. Now it is time to begin trimming the clerical and support staff to prepare for the new system. There are 250 positions that will have to be abolished in the first stage of the process. Although some transitional dollars are available to assist those who will lose their positions, the funds will be too little and too late to provide a smooth transition. Employees are going to be hurt. Separation packages will be skinny.

Operational planning sessions have been under way for weeks and the management structure is showing signs of severe stress. Your senior associate drops by late one afternoon and casually hands you an envelope containing her letter of resignation. She looks depressed and simply says that she cannot take the pressure anymore: the job simply isn't worth it. She has accepted a position in the hotel field. You take this as devastating news since she has been one of the key members of the team and you were counting on her to help ease the organization through the crisis.

That night you do some very serious thinking about your capacity to lead. Are others preparing to bail out? What immediate steps could be taken to inspire the management team so the depression you are feeling will not be communicated to others? If you hadn't recognized it before, you do now. Leadership is not without its costs. All of your training and experience is about to be tested as never before.

Somehow the challenge inspires you; you realize you are up to the task. The health care system is broken and you want to be a crucial partner in the process of fixing it. This is the theme that you carry forth and communicate to your staff in the days and months to come.

It is clear now that the whole health care system is going to have to be fixed. Young families face bankruptcy because of the prohibitive costs of health insurance. Capitation plans (HMOs) cannot produce a solution because patients who are considered poor risks are being gradually eliminated from coverage. The elderly are rebelling as the portion of their medical bill covered by insurance steadily declines. The Medicaid system is seriously underfunded. And the administrative costs associated with such a fragmented system are unmanageable. An incremental approach to change will be too little and too late.

Regardless of when and what type of reform is implemented, the impact will be substantial. Executives who are ten or more years from retirement will have to brave the storm and be ready to adapt when the time comes to make significant changes. It is important to start anticipating what the new millenium will bring and to plan to do what we can to adapt to and embrace the new system.

Reorienting Health Care Executives

As the current system gradually gets phased out, regardless of the type of system that gets phased in, health care executives will be forced to reexamine much of what they do. New skills and a new orientation will be essential to manage and lead in the new era. Reforms are certain to affect at least three areas of concern to health care leaders: management priorities and technical expertise, the executive's social responsibility, and executive leadership style. This chapter will focus on specific changes that are likely to come about in the health care environment and the specific ways in which health care leaders will be called upon to respond to them.

Changes in Management Priorities and Technical Expertise

Information systems. Under any new system of health care delivery, one of the first areas that executives will have to address is the upgrading of data and information systems, initially to aid in understanding and implementing the internal operating systems that would be needed under new payer systems, but ultimately to identify the true costs of producing services and to establish budget controls based on an effective cost-driven base.

Preparation for change in information systems has to include the upgrading of the organization's knowledge about the power and use of new technology. A capable information systems team will have to be in place to engineer the linking of new payer systems and the accurate collection of data, and to promote the application of systems thinking in decision making. This means that leaders must become more involved in tracking technology, and in order to manage the overall institutional approach, we must all become computer literate.

Financial control. Because of their experience with DRGs, hospitals will have a head start over group practices when tracking resource consumption. Executives have already been forced to shift the composition of their management teams to include more staff with the capacity to work on budgeting, forecasting, and cost control. This will allow them to adapt to a new system in which organizations contract directly with employers to provide health services under the health benefit standards established by the federal government.

But group practice executives will need to link up with their hospital counterparts to participate in the contracting process. The health care system of the future will not be free of competition: the single payer approach will seek to reduce expenses through intersystem bidding for market share. Efficient providers will be rewarded, and those who are less efficient will be penalized. The system will protect isolated providers (for example, in rural communities), but linkages demonstrating financial control capacity will be especially protected (for example, urban-rural linkages).

Human resources. In addition to increasing the team's knowledge base about information systems and finances, the health care executive of the year 2000 will need to be much more sensitive to the management of human resources. If events unfold as predicted, shortages of professionals in almost every classification will mean that management will need to be proficient in creating organizational environments that attract and retain these professionals. The role of the human resources director will be vastly enhanced in the organizational structure. Leaders should consider giving special human resources training to executives who have been functioning in line positions and who are knowledgeable about working conditions on the front line. Once they have received the proper training, these managers could be placed in full-time human resources activities.

Patient services. Changes in the health care system are likely to bring about changes in the way organizations approach patient services. If patients are allowed to choose which regional health system they wish to use, providers will become aware that, to retain volume and maintain the viability of the system, they must give more attention to satisfying patient needs. All organizations would need trained staff assigned as ombudsmen to quickly resolve patient or family concerns—a difficult task since health care providers would be serving more patients and operating under significant resource constraints. Executives would then spend more time ensuring that quality-of-care mechanisms are effective and that they relate closely to patient expectations of service.

Leaders must begin immediately to stress their organization's focus on service. We need to initiate systems to provide rapid feedback on the satisfaction levels of patients served, and we need to foster new attitudes to counter any perception that the individual does not matter under the new system. Continuous quality improvement programs should be a top priority.

Systems orientation. A new system emphasizing integrated care would need leadership from executives who have a systems orientation to health care delivery, as contrasted with a single organizational or institutional orientation. If all systems were not only internally integrated but also closely linked with public health agencies having a vastly expanded role in preventive medicine, executives would need to be much more knowledgeable about public health care activities. Leaders can and should anticipate that they will need to function as strategic executives in the future, and they should try to acquire knowledge about how the various elements of the health care system might fit together to provide high-quality care to the patient.

Marketing and promotion. It seems likely that, under a national health plan emphasizing coverage of basic services, marketing to patients would begin to focus on two primary audiences: the potential enrollee and the affluent consumer. The potential enrollee to the regional health system would be the target of marketing that attempts to demonstrate quality and responsiveness to patient needs, as contrasted with the medical and surgical specialty marketing that has been so common recently. The second audience would be the citizen who has elected to pay substantially higher out-of-pocket premiums for coverage of special services. The health care executive would have to pay close attention to the perceived quality of service that the affluent consumer receives because, for the high fees necessary to acquire that service, the patient's expectations would be very high. Under such a system, the extra revenue from these patients would be essential to the operation of resource-constrained regional health systems.

If this dual patient-service concept (in which all citizens would be enrolled and affluent patients would be allowed to pay for extra services) were adopted, the leader would face a new challenge. Under the current system, professionals adhere to processes that attempt to minimize service discrimination based on the level or type of an individual's insurance coverage. Yet we all know that such discrimination occurs. The system of the future may actually require differentiation. The patient insured under a basic plan may not have access to the ultimate in service. The challenge to the health care executive would be to manage these dual systems of service—particularly the personal service aspect of the care—under the same organizational roof. The leader would have to seriously consider how to adapt the culture of the delivery organization to these new value system requirements.

Changes in the Executive's Social Responsibility

Advocating change. Health care executives are going to find themselves increasingly in the public eye. As the health system breaks down under the weight of its accumulated problems (aging population, federal budget problems, and access issues), the role of the health care executive as a spokesperson will assume more importance. Perhaps executives will begin by trying to justify what is taking place, to protect the status quo, or to minimize the shock that change will bring to the organization. But eventually leaders will need to become proactive advocates for change. Health care leaders should start now by making an investment in additional training to further develop communication skills and by spending more time on networking with community leaders and others to increase public understanding of health policy issues.

Interacting at the local level. Although professional societies and health industry associations will continue to play a significant role in monitoring and stimulating useful change, the lack of a truly unbiased forum for national debate means that health care leaders will need to become much more visible and articulate on health issues at the local level. Executives will focus less on addressing the interests of single organizations than on resolving public health issues such as disease prevention, improved home care, and so on. For executives who have been wrapped up in managing the internal affairs of their organizations, and who are devoting relatively little effort to outside issues, this change will take a major shift in orientation.

Getting involved in bioethics. As the courts get closer to resolving basic issues such as those relating to the right to die (and even conflict over the right to life versus free choice relating to abortion), the implications for bioethics will assume increasing importance. The technical competence of professionals and the advancement of science and technology will continue to raise new questions about matters such as the manipulation of human genes to improve resistance to chronic diseases. Scientists will push to further improve the quality and longevity of life through the rearrangement of genetic structures, and their research will eventually force us to face the question of how much is enough.

In addition, as organ and body part transplants become more common, the health care executive, along with others, will face the new and ever more complicated assignment of trying to determine what the responsibility of the health services organization should be in response to these new and provocative solutions to the prevention of disease and the treatment of chronic disease. The sheer cost of these procedures will cause the acceleration of the debate on rationing of care. Bioethics should be on health care leaders' list of priorities, and executives should work on becoming more knowledgeable about the legal and moral implications of bioethical issues.

Changes in Leadership Style

Under a national health system, leaders would probably preside over flat, democratic, consensus-building structures staffed with qualified management and professional specialists who would be trained to work as unified teams. Organizations would be linked into significant regional systems involving all components (from rural units emphasizing emergency and preventive care to tertiary care centers), and encompassing hospice, home health care, and skilled nursing services as well. If such a system is implemented, the health care executive might function as a "minister of health" over these systems and would need management tools that work to build and maintain the focus of the organization through consensus and teamwork.

Regardless of the type of system that is implemented, one of the most powerful tools at the executive's disposal will be his or her capacity to negotiate relationships with payers (in the case of national health insurance, this means the government). The ability to function as a health care diplomat, ensuring the integration of health services for the common good of the citizen, will be of paramount importance.

Senior executives in the year 2000 will need to supplement their skill in financial affairs with more general skills. The generalist background will help the executive approach complicated issues with a well-rounded but unbiased viewpoint. Intellectual creativity and the ability to compromise to bring closure to problems will be much in demand by boards of regional health care organizations. Health care executives will need to be comfortable with their role and recognize that they must depend on their specialist teams to deal with the operational issues—and they will need to trust their colleagues to be inventive in doing so. The leader will have to build a well-rounded team that includes physicians who are schooled in the administrative and managerial sciences. And the leader will have to be charismatic enough to pull together the various professional components involved in health care delivery to work toward a common cause.

Conclusion

Of course, many of the characteristics of excellent leadership today will continue to be useful under any new system. Basic adherence to strict ethical codes and values will be essential. Skill in motivating others will always be high on the list. The ability to take a low profile to accomplish strategic goals rather than asserting an ego-oriented management style will still be most productive. Time for teaching and mentoring should be part of the leader's commitment to health care.

The best advice for the leader who wishes to make a difference is to devote time and thought to the constant tuning of his or her professional skills. The road may be uncertain at times, but if you possess and retain the belief that you can make a difference, you will vastly improve your chances of achieving all of your personal and professional objectives.

15

THE BIG PICTURE:
A CALL FOR NATIONAL LEADERSHIP

"Would you tell me, please, which way I ought to go from here?"
"That depends a good deal on where you want to get to," said the Cat.
"I don't much care where—" said Alice.
"Then it doesn't matter which way you go," said the Cat.

Lewis Carroll, *Alice's Adventures in Wonderland*

Nearly everyone can offer a fix for an isolated issue in health care, whether the issue is increasing access, controlling costs, dealing with AIDS, or improving the overall health of our citizens. But nobody seems to agree about the best way to cure the system itself. We are floundering in the absence of consensus on a single national health policy. The major debate has shifted from whether or not we need to improve the health system to what form the change should take and when it should occur. Will it be national in scope or state managed, or should we engage in what might be termed "raging incrementalism"—picking at pieces of the problem without ever addressing the whole?

The extraordinary political changes that have occurred in recent years throughout the world, beginning with the fall of the Berlin Wall in 1989, have led some analysts to suggest that a peace dividend could be declared

Portions of this chapter have been adapted, with the permission of The Society of Thoracic Surgeons, from A. Ross, "The Perspective of the Industry," *Annals of Thoracic Surgery* 52, no. 2 (1991): 385–89.

that would infuse the existing health system with substantial new funds. However, the war in the Persian Gulf, the continuing unrest in the Middle East, and the growing national debt and deepening recession in the United States have quickly squelched any remaining optimism about the possibility of a peace dividend. The national deficit problems are so severe and the national infrastructure (particularly education, transportation, and the environment) is so in need of repair that it seems unlikely that health care will be the major recipient of any largesse. More likely, in fact, is the possibility that budget pressures will force new rounds of cutbacks in funds for health services. It now appears that the only way to increase equitable access to care and control costs will be through some kind of nationally mandated system for health care.

Even so, resistance to a national health plan seems deeply rooted. Perhaps we have become so familiar with disorder and inequity that we are more comfortable with them than with change. As Stephen Shortell and Walter McNerney stated, "It would be tempting to suggest that the U.S. health care system is now in disarray were it not for the fact that it has never been otherwise."[1] But this disarray is not caused by a lack of proposals for new initiatives. Rather, our lack of consensus is woven into the cultural and societal fabric of our multifaceted society.

Our population is not homogeneous, and this detracts from the ability of a single political group to force system change. The labor movement, for example, is much weaker in the United States than it is in Europe. In addition, diverse taxing structures in the states and in the federal system, combined with the reluctance of our citizens to vote in new taxes, make it difficult for legislators to mandate new basic health care benefits.

Finally, the paranoia that accompanies the imposition of regulations on business carries over into health care, where competition between health care providers has been encouraged as a national policy (at least until recently). Such competition tends to slow down the creation of cooperative ventures and networks between health care providers, which in turn makes it more difficult to build a health policy consensus among providers. (In fact, antitrust issues are suggested as a means of discouraging mergers between health care providers, in spite of the fact that, if permitted, mergers might favorably affect the health of citizens.) At the microfinancial level, the practice of allowing employers to deduct health insurance premium expenses as a business expense has the effect of delaying the need to incorporate health insurance costs into a universally applied tax base. Many of those citizens who are uninsured are employed by small businesses that elect not to provide insurance coverage, or that elect to employ many part-time employees as a means of reducing business expenses.

The discussion over the pros and cons of a national system for health care has been going on for some time now. Whether or not the concept of a national plan for health care appeals to you or not may well depend on your particular situation. Executives in well-positioned health services organizations that are experiencing a solid bottom line may be more likely to find the scenario depressing. But if one supports the concept that basic health care must be available to all citizens regardless of their ability to pay, then this forecast may be more acceptable. Even those of us who are well insured do not have to look far to find aging parents, relatives, or close friends who, because they are marginally employed with minimal or no health insurance coverage, are poorly equipped to handle catastrophic health care costs. When you witness the erosion of their coverage it seems obvious that change is inevitable.

Perspectives on National Health Care

The major motive for embarking on a national health program in the United States traditionally has been concern for health care costs, which is not as strong a rallying point politically as is concern for the societal inequities that occur without a national health policy. There is, however, growing concern about the number of Americans who do not have adequate health insurance protection and are vulnerable in times of medical need. Citizens are beginning to understand the need and the complexity of the problem, so traditional alliances do seem to be changing. The alliances on health issues between business and health care providers, and between labor and government, are different now than they were even a few years ago.

David Kinzer, who for many years was the president of the Massachusetts Hospital Association and more recently was a professor at the Harvard University School of Public Health, was viewed by health care executives as one of the brightest and best health theorists in the land. In 1990, he wrote in *The New England Journal of Medicine* that the problem with health care in the United States is "pluralism itself, which many of our health care leaders seem to think must be retained at all costs. There is a deeply imbedded conviction that the only way to protect health providers against too much government control is to keep all escape hatches open."[2] Whether we represent labor, government, providers, or others, we must make some concessions to work toward building a national consensus that will address this multifaceted problem. The end result will not be business as usual, and we must grow to accept that.

At the American Hospital Association meeting in July of 1990, former U.S. Surgeon General C. Everett Koop said, "In a word, we have big problems." He commented facetiously that he had considered issuing a health bulletin to read, "Warning: The Surgeon General has determined that the health care system might be detrimental to your health." On the other hand, Koop warned against the implementation of a national health program, noting that national health care is based on "planned scarcity." Such a system, he said, ultimately results in an erosion of quality, productivity, and responsiveness, and can lead to health care rationing.[3] It is interesting to note, however, that in many ways the system we have is already based on rationing—rationing based on personal economic status.

Another respected spokesperson for health care policy, Arnold Relman, issued a call to the medical profession in 1989 in which he said, "Physicians will have to play an active and constructive part in shaping the new health care system, because no comprehensive arrangement is likely to succeed without their cooperation." Relman stated that "now is the time for our profession to make common cause with government and with the major private payers in seeking solutions to a pressing social problem that is not going to solve itself."[4] But the pathway to achieving common cause is torturous indeed.

Relman should be very pleased with the position taken recently by the American College of Physicians, which called for the development of a single national health policy to resolve the health care needs of the nation. This unexpected action taken by a large professional organization caught many by surprise, but it also served to transmit the message to the American public that physicians too are concerned. It is an encouraging sign that one of the largest professional societies in the nation has taken such a step. It appears to be a signal that some are moving away from postures of incremental change to positions that offer the potential of aiding in the process of building a new national consensus.

In spite of growing agitation, there has not been much accomplished nationally toward the development of a new policy. The Pepper Commission attempted a solution but ultimately was divided in its support for the recommendations it made in its report.[5] The Pepper Commission recommended extending coverage to the 31,000,000 uninsured Americans through a combination of public and private initiatives. Although this program had a lot going for it, seven of the fifteen members of the bipartisan commission who labored so diligently voted against the final recommendations of the panel.

Nor did the National Leadership Commission on Health Care, another ad hoc bipartisan commission, resolve the problem. There were simply too many divergent viewpoints that made it impractical to build an action-oriented consensus. Unfortunately, it appears that the only way a consensus will develop is if the health care crisis worsens to the point that individual agendas become less important than public and private pressure for reform.

A Unified Vision of the Future

Perhaps these commissions failed because of the lack of commitment to a common vision. As a nation, we seem to continue to approach health problems incrementally rather than establishing a unified perspective and common goal. We isolate key facts and symptoms, and in the best American tradition, we work toward a quick fix. We do so in a health care environment in which the clinical team consists of a group of individuals, each of whom has a unique and different agenda and something to protect.

It is very difficult to resolve issues when the parties around the table bring predetermined goals and are accountable to others who set their agenda from a distance. This, of course, is in keeping with our grand old American tradition of "minding the store" and keeping in touch with our constituents. If a bit more untethered, the participants in the policymaking process might agree to recommend solutions that would produce significant results. But unfortunately, we are continuing to focus on short-range concerns and we are dealing with them as isolated events. Catastrophic health care is a notable example. Cost containment is another. Physician payment reform is a third example. Many people assume that resolving these three separate issues, along with many others, can produce an organized, synchronized, and integrated health services program. But such wishful thinking seems absurd.

Ed Connors, president of Mercy Health Services and 1989 chair of the American Hospital Association, has suggested that we need to fund and support an existing organization, which is known for its nonpartisan approaches to problems and has already demonstrated cohesion as a group, to work on addressing the overall picture of health care delivery in the United States.[6] We should pour in government dollars, seek out foundations for support, pull in business contributions, and draw heavily from the health sector as well. Connors suggests that the ideal organization to accept this task is the Institute of Medicine because it is well led, has national credibility, and has demonstrated its fund-raising abilities. It has a culture and history, and cohesive participants who function in the interest of the common good.

Whatever the group, if it is to succeed it must be untainted with special interests. It must be an organization with a track record of working together toward the public good. (Think about your own nominee for such an awesome task—it must be able both to recommend a national health policy and to hammer out a national consensus.) Unfortunately, few such organizations come to mind, and that is precisely the dilemma. A new commission of even the most well-intentioned people, if it lacks the history and experience of working together and represents totally diverse interests, has too great a challenge on its hands.

What Stands in the Way?

Whoever does take on the task of reforming the health care system will
have to contend with a number of obstacles. It is not just how and when to
get there that poses a problem. Before any group or organization bring the
nation to any kind of unified vision, it will face a multitude of conflicting
issues, interests, and options, of which those outlined below are only a few.

Diverse Issues

The most frustrating aspect of all of this is that, in the absence of reform,
we find a growing list of critical issues that need to be dealt with if we are
to do right by our patients. The longer we wait to reform the system, the
more severe the issues become and the more policymakers feel the pressure
from every direction.

Access. The issue of access is critical. More than any other single issue,
this will be the one most likely to force health system reform. With some
34 million citizens finding it difficult or impossible to get access to health
care, the crisis is clearly mounting. Although the Medicaid programs provide
some basic support for the truly poor, those who are at or above the poverty
line have been ignored.

Families who do not have coverage through employers—particularly
young families who also do not have high incomes or sizable savings
accounts—find it impossible to obtain affordable insurance, so they are
forced to go without coverage. One catastrophic health experience can easily
lead to personal bankruptcy, and in fact, the rate of personal bankruptcy in
the United States is already rapidly on the rise, particularly among young
Americans.

Because insurance companies are struggling to control the rate of increase of their premiums, they are excluding employee groups from coverage
if a group's experience rating declines because of higher utilization of health
care services. Small companies, unable to maintain health insurance coverage because of increasing premium costs, are shifting premium increases to
employees or are eliminating coverage altogether as a means of maintaining
their economic survival.

Medicare beneficiaries are realizing that the government is paying
fewer cents on the dollar than ever before for health care charges. As a
result, they face high premium costs for supplemental coverage for routine
services or for protection against the economic hazards of being placed in a
nursing home.

Bioethics. Solving bioethical questions, particularly with regard to the use of technology, is also still ahead of us. For example, the technology for performing organ transplants has now exceeded our capacity to find organ donors. We have come a long way since the days when anonymous panels had to select patients to go on renal dialysis, all the while knowing that without the dialysis the other patients would certainly die. But the issues are still the same. Should the ultimate decision about whether or not to perform a bone marrow transplant rest on the patient's capacity to pay the bill? Is it reasonable to expect hospitals to care for all patients presenting themselves for nonemergency care, at the expense of full-paying patients? These and other issues are very difficult to solve, but it is clear that rationing of health care is taking place under the present system (based on insurance or resource coverage). The compelling argument for implementing national reform of the health care system is that rationing of care based on the individual's capacity to pay would be minimized.

Litigation. We have been floundering with tort reform issues for decades. Even in California, where tort reforms have been excellent, the time line for implementing the reforms was lengthy. Since the reforms, however, California's medical liability premiums have been stable. Among other changes, the reduction in the statute of limitations and the capping of awards for pain and suffering have helped to create a stable insurance market in a state that previously had experienced rapidly spiraling rates. Despite the time it has taken, the experience in California should be an indication that solutions are possible.

What we need now, though, is a national solution to the problem of excess litigation. No one objects to providing reasonable compensation for true damage, but the propensity of the American citizen to look for someone to blame and then to sue has to be bridled. Perhaps you recall the case where a woman whose child was impaired as a result of her alcoholism sued the liquor manufacturer for the damage that alcohol caused to the fetus. The fact that the mother lost the case is beside the point. The point is that tort reform is desperately needed but little progress is being made.

Education and research. The cutbacks by the federal government on funding of medical education have been relatively modest so far, but there are indications that they will get worse. Auditing is under way in many teaching hospitals, which suggests that new base lines are going to be developed. At some point, some of our preeminent medical training sites may find themselves unable to maintain the same quality of teaching that they had in the past. A shifting of financing mechanisms away from support of both medical education and research will erode the high quality of medicine in this nation.

These interrelated but distinctly different issues all bear on the quality of patient care and all need resolution, and we can spend unlimited energy as providers on any one of them. But if we solve these issues independently, as opposed to finding a way to pull together a national consensus and address the issues as a total package, we will not do well for our patients or for ourselves.

Diverse Interests

It is difficult to arrive at a national consensus with so many factions involved in the debate. When we look at the health care system as a whole and think about what systematic reforms would resolve the greatest number of problems, the diverse and complex interests involved in reform become apparent.

Labor. Labor representatives are not eager to see employers push benefit costs back to the employee through the imposition of increasing co-deductibles or reduction of dependent coverage. Representatives of labor are also not interested in having employers limit coverage just to the lowest cost provider. Quality of care is important, too. Unions representing employees who work in plants and businesses that cross state boundaries do not want to support fragmented local option solutions to health care reform, so they look for national strategies as a solution.

Employers. Employers deplore the rapid increase in health care premiums because of the impact that premiums have on their cost structure, but employers also seem to fight the concept of any mandatory basic health insurance coverage at employer expense, even though such legislation might help stabilize premiums and reduce cost shifting. Some employers, particularly small businesses, are currently transferring portions of premium costs to their employees, in some cases as a matter of financial survival. The most attractive solution to future funding of health care seems to be a broad-based change in the tax structure to help spread costs widely rather than using special purpose tax increases aimed just at the business community.

Tax payers. Tax payers with health insurance coverage do not want taxes to be raised but seem to believe that it is their absolute right to have access to all health services, elective as well as urgent, in a timely fashion. And many patients seem to feel that if the outcome is not up to their expectations, then suing is the only answer. They take the attitude that if something goes wrong, somebody must be to blame. The only meaningful solution to the current epidemic of litigation is meaningful tort reform on a national basis.

Elected officials. Elected officials at all levels abhor the unpredictable nature of health care cost increases. They address the problem politically by cutting back on legitimate and much needed government payments to hospitals, physicians, and others. They recognize that voters want change as long as it does not affect them personally. Elected officials abhor increases in the cost of health services, particularly when they are facing so many other legitimate demands for aid (for example, for education, housing, transportation, and the environment). But what really puts the pressure on them is the rapidity and unpredictability of the escalation of costs. Predictability is essential if there is to be a balanced budget. At some magic moment, sooner rather than later, the constituent pressure for reform will outweigh the inertia associated with normal political processes and elected officials will receive a virtual mandate to proceed with system reform.

The medical community. Finally, how does the medical establishment address the problem? What signposts do we put up to help direct our colleagues and consumers through the "wonderland" of health care? In the past we have been opposed to a lot of the proposed changes. We tend to oppose cutbacks in the budget but we want to invest more in new construction and technology. We fight intramurally and quite frequently appear to be politically fragmented—and most tragically, we do so for reasons that are perceived to be self-serving. Many of our initiatives seem to be taken to protect our revenue and profits, both of which are legitimate concerns, but we do not always pull together effectively when speaking out on key issues such as access, litigation, education and research support, and others. Nor do we speak as a unified group on issues of preventive medicine, mental health, or the need to address the very real issues of technology assessment, rationing of care, and the other bioethical issues of the day.

Still, many of us do see things that are going right. Among them are the following:

- Breakthroughs in research
- The development of new technology that is the best in the world
- The development of integrated systems of care linking urban, suburban, and rural hospitals
- Service to provide continuity of care
- The move away from hospitalization into the ambulatory setting, not just for cost-containment purposes but for attacking health problems before hospitalization becomes necessary
- The recognition of the importance of primary care

- Willingness on the part of physicians to include other professionals in the team in managing patient care

- Improved quality of management

- The use of data banks and computers to validate results and to work effectively on quality issues within the institutional setting without waiting for those federal data banks to force change

- Willingness on the part of organizations to take public stands proactively on controversial issues

- The gradual recognition by industry, which tends to approach health care as a cost-cutting exercise, of the complexity of health delivery

- The fragmentation of traditional alliances, which will mix things up and could potentially bring together a greater understanding and consensus on problems

- Growing willingness on the part of physicians to become involved in supporting programs that broaden viewpoints toward health, combined with a recognition that problems can no longer be solved incrementally and in small bites

So where does all this lead us? Remembering that there are few simple solutions to complex problems, what is to be done for the good of the common cause? Do we have reason to hope that things will get better, or is the problem so large that it is beyond resolution until events create a genuine crisis? And what should health care providers be doing other than wringing their hands and fighting short-range skirmishes?

Diverse Options

Perhaps a little history will help. Remember the dire forecast associated with the passage of Medicare—that the end was in sight, that Medicare would be the beginning of socialized medicine and the end of the quality of medicine. It did not quite turn out that way. Even with all its frustrations (for both providers and patients), the program worked. As providers we may complain about poor fee schedules, but before Medicare and Medicaid, many patients without resources received charity care or went without. The point is that although we do not yet have the best solution, we should continue to seek one out. And we do have a few examples of programs that, although not flawless, are addressing some of the critical issues.

The Oregon approach. The state of Oregon, through legislative action creating the Basic Health Services Act of Oregon, has approached the issue of containing health care costs through a program of rationing of care on the basis of need. (The act currently applies only to Medicaid patients.) The plan employs medical and surgical procedure lists to establish funding priorities. For example, certain organ transplants would be significantly limited in order to provide more financial support for preventive medicine or prenatal care. End-stage AIDS patients would receive less support than those beneficiaries who could recover completely with treatment. Limited funding of intensive care for the elderly would leave more funds available for trauma systems.

The Oregon plan is an innovative but controversial method of addressing a serious problem, that is, determining the best way to allocate diminishing resources. The system represents a cost-benefit analysis approach to rationing health care. Although it is certainly a viable road to take, it is not one that will settle very easily if ultimately applied to the middle-income and affluent citizenry of Oregon. We could even expect a migration of some citizens from Oregon to other states because of the limitations, which points out one of the hazards of a state-by-state approach to health care reform. But the Oregon approach bears watching. Representatives of other states, the federal government, businesses, and ethicists will all be monitoring the program very carefully.

The Canadian system. Although the Canadian provinces differ from one another, the costs of care are theoretically controlled through budget negotiating among the three primary players—the Ministry of Health, physicians, and hospitals—on a province-by-province basis. Of course, elective care is also allocated in part through queuing. The patient may wait for beds, physician specialty services, and lots of other things, but the total process produces reasonably predictable health care costs, which is what government and businesses seek.

Note also that the Canadian health system applies to all. It may have some problems, but it cannot be faulted for failing to provide access to those who are in need. For instance, in 1990 the waiting line became too long for elective bypass surgery in British Columbia, and the British Columbia Minister of Health elected to purchase these services from hospitals in the United States. In this instance, hospitals in the state of Washington were asked to bid to provide bypass surgery. Two hospitals in Seattle were initially selected: the University of Washington and Virginia Mason Medical Center. So although the patients were not able to receive the surgery within the Canadian system, the provincial government did arrange for and purchase the needed services. In contrast, how would uninsured citizens in the United States find timely access to elective bypass surgery?

A policy of no change. There is at least one alternative to developing a full-stage program, which is to make no significant change except in small increments. And there are some who say that is the way to go, that lots of things are working well and we should not tinker with the system too much or too fast. Unfortunately, the pace is building and those who advocate no change will find themselves left behind. More and more cities will find that they are becoming communities filled with contrasts. Seattle has some hospitals on the edge of the city that are showing significant profits. Downtown hospitals, on the other hand, are carrying more nonpaying or partially paying patients, and as they contend with the issue of how to pay for care for drug-addicted patients, the elderly, and the mentally ill, they are beginning to struggle just as hospitals do in other urban areas. An unbalanced system in a single city suggests that the problem is astounding on a national scale.

Stepping Up the Pace of Change

When federal data banks begin to produce their figures, display the outcome results for every physician by procedure, and then publish this information, we are likely to see an explosive reaction, which will be followed by an accelerated investment by hospitals and physicians in further developing their data systems to monitor results more closely. Ironically, whether or not this information is accurate, it will probably be the release of the data nationally that will spur us on to action—action that we might not otherwise have taken and that, so far, we seem to be avoiding.

The Challenge to Leaders

We are on the verge of a change in the health care system that is going to affect hospitals, physicians, and providers. The end result, after a shakedown period, will have to be acceptable to both patients and providers. What needs to be done, of course, is for all parties to work toward consensus on major policy issues by addressing the following questions:

1. How will the new program be funded and structured? Should payments be based on performance?
2. Will it be state based and federally integrated?
3. How will the volume of services be controlled?
4. Will there be a single benefit level for all, or will it be possible for some to go outside the system at personal expense? Is this good or bad?

5. Will the new program be implemented in stages rather than in one enormous step?

6. What role should health services executives, physicians, and other providers play in the scheme of things?

7. What forum or body can be found to help build the consensus so desperately needed to ensure a new and fairer system?

The contemporary health care executive is really at a crossroads where tough choices will have to be made. One road leads to a course of behavior that will attempt to preserve the status quo, to minimize the speed of change and protect traditional practices and values. The other road leads to encouraging and embracing change by actively structuring systems to meet new environmental and organizational needs. The leader will take the second trail, embracing change and anticipating the way environmental changes will affect the organization. This does not mean that old values are discarded or that organizations should be disrupted with premature forecasts of doom. Instead, it means that thoughtful preparation—a review of what works best and an inventory of what might need strengthening—will be needed.

The process of preparing organizations for change is a long one, and because it requires the participation of the organization's many stakeholders, it cannot be embarked upon singlehandedly. The leader should reflect on these points when working up an organizational strategy for ensuring continued success:

1. Accept the fact that fewer resources will be available to do more work. Human resources will need to be carefully analyzed to ensure that the right mix of managers and staff have been recruited and integrated into close-knit and highly effective teams. It is essential to avoid turnover among key players in the midst of change. When a new national health system is actually being implemented, leaders will have no time to think about team mix and function. These issues need to be addressed well in advance of systemwide changes.

2. Recognize that the organization of the future will not look like today's typical organization. It will be significantly reshaped. Leading organizations are already eliminating layers of management and working diligently to balance the need for control with the need to promote decentralization in decision making. The organization best equipped for the future will be even flatter in structure. As a result, it may be necessary for the leader to develop an entirely new management style. For example, instead of controlling decision making from the top, leaders will have to reprogram themselves to trust

subordinates more and to provide much more latitude in decision making to physicians, nurses, managers, and other professionals. This also means that leaders and others in the organization will have to accept a certain amount of chaos as controls are transferred from one level in the organization to another.

3. Allocate additional resources to strategic planning. Since even subtle shifts in national policy could have a profound effect on individual organizations, leaders will need to anticipate the impact. Strategic planning will change from being a separate function in the organization to being highly integrated into operational decision making. Product or service line managers, for example, will need continual access to planning disciplines to provide state-of-the-art use of data and forecasting technology.

4. Learn to cope with conflicts of personal and organizational values and ethics. As old ways are modified, leaders will have to help diffuse the tension that accompanies change. Physicians, for example, will face trying times as incomes are constrained through the implementation of controlled fee schedules. Such constraints might place the physicians in an adversarial position with hospitals as revenue is capped for both groups. Leaders must anticipate such conflicts and build systems that help bind stakeholders together in a common cause.

   In addition, as organizational and personal innovation is encouraged, leaders must monitor behavior patterns on a systemwide basis to ensure that innovation is not used by some as a justification for abandoning ethical practices. In fact, leaders need to foster the development of written statements that define in broad terms what constitutes appropriate behavior. (An example of such a statement can be found in Chapter 2).

5. Actively prepare a strategy to minimize the potential for erosion of performance within the organization. As units are stressed by the elimination of traditional support systems under financial constraints, there will be a tendency to cut corners, to let things drift, and to blame things on the fact that there is too much to do. Leaders must anticipate this and put into motion programs that enrich the work environment by freeing up the individual to participate in important projects. Obviously, those who have invested time and energy in establishing well-grounded programs in continuous quality improvement will be well positioned to minimize the erosion of performance.

Conclusion

As leaders, we need to focus our efforts on promoting the need for change, and to work diligently to focus public and governmental attention on the choices that are still ahead of us. If we elect to sit on the sidelines and hope for a return to the days of old, or worse yet, function like the Cheshire Cat by offering seemingly profound advice that actually is meaningless, we will reap rewards of the same significance.

Notes

1. S. M. Shortell and W. J. McNerney, "Criteria and Guidelines for Reforming the U.S. Health Care System," *New England Journal of Medicine* 322, no. 7 (1990): 463–67.
2. D. Kinzer, "Universal Entitlement to Health Care," *New England Journal of Medicine* 322, no. 7 (1990): 468–70.
3. C. E. Koop, "Keynote Address," *American Hospital Association News* 26, no. 29 (1990): 2.
4. A. Relman, "Universal Health Insurance: Its Time Has Come," *New England Journal of Medicine* 320, no. 2 (1989): 117–18.
5. The Pepper Commission, "A Call to Action," Final Report of the U.S. Bipartisan Commission on Comprehensive Health Care (Washington, DC: U.S. Government Printing Office, 1990).
6. E. Connors, "Reflections on Leadership in Health Care: A Conversation with Edward J. Connors," *Hospital & Health Services Administration* 35, no. 3 (1990): 309–20.

EPILOGUE

When all is said and done, what is this leadership business all about? The acid test of success is not necessarily whether the health care organization has grown in size or whether the bottom line is predictably in the black. Some of the best leaders have been willing to enter failing organizations that were needed in their community, but they may *not* have succeeded in turning the organizations around. Success is not always measured by the achievement of a goal. Sometimes it is measured by an individual's courage to make a difference, and this is true at any level in an organization.

Nor is success always measured in dollars, contrary to the opinion of many. Some leaders have given up prestigious positions to accept the challenge of putting together a new community service. They were not concerned that some of their colleagues thought that they had lost the game. The question of what defines success can only be answered by the individual. It is a personal event.

Some leaders feel a sense of destiny, which gives them a level of self-confidence that carries them through the tough times. They may not fully understand their motivation, but they know they can make a difference. For others, the process is more difficult but just as rewarding. They craft their skills carefully, enhancing their leadership knowledge through diligent effort and hard work. They control their egos, learn to observe and adapt, and do not leap to precipitous judgments concerning either people or issues. They make mistakes and then try to improve. They constantly adapt, and so they succeed. Ultimately, leadership success has to be measured in very personal terms. Do you believe that you have made a difference in improving your organization? If so, you have succeeded.

SUGGESTED READINGS

Allcorn, S. "Using Matrix Organization to Manage Health Care Delivery Organizations." *Hospital & Health Services Administration* 35, no. 4 (1990): 575–90.

Applegate, L. M., et al. "Information Technology and Tomorrow's Manager." *Harvard Business Review* 66, no. 6 (1988): 128–32.

Bartlett, C. A., and S. Ghoshal. "Matrix Management: Not a Structure, a Frame of Mind." *Harvard Business Review* 68, no. 4 (1990): 138–45.

Bennis, W., and B. Nanus. *Leaders: The Strategies for Taking Charge.* New York: Harper & Row, 1985.

Berwick, D. "Continuous Improvement as an Ideal in Health Care." *New England Journal of Medicine* 320, no. 1 (1989): 53–56.

Bigelow, B., and J. F. Mahon. "Strategic Behavior of Hospitals: A Framework for Analysis." *Medical Care Review* 46, no. 3 (1989): 295–311.

Bowers, M. R. "Product Line Management in Hospitals: An Exploratory Study of Managing Change." *Hospital & Health Services Administration* 35, no. 3 (1990): 365–75.

Boyle, R. "Failure Avoidance: Will You Be Singing in the Rain?" *Healthcare Forum Journal* 31, no. 5 (1988): 10–18.

Brown, M., and B. P. McCool. "Health Care Systems: Predictions for the Future." *Health Care Management Review* 15, no. 3 (1990): 87–94.

Burns, J. M. *Leadership.* New York: Harper & Row, 1978.

Conrad, D. A., and W. L. Dowling. "Vertical Integration in Health Care Services: Theory and Managerial Implications." *Health Care Management Review* 15, no. 4 (1990): 9–22.

Darr, K., B. Longest, Jr., and J. Rakich. "The Ethical Imperative in Health Services Governance and Management." *Hospital & Health Services Administration* 31, no. 2 (1986): 53–66.

Deal, T. "Healthcare Executives as Symbolic Leaders." *Healthcare Executive* 5, no. 2 (1990): 24–27.

Deal, T., and A. Kennedy. *Corporate Cultures.* Reading, MA: Addison-Wesley, 1982.

Drucker, P. F. "What Business Can Learn from Nonprofits." *Harvard Business Review* 67, no. 4 (1989): 88–93.

Etzioni, A. "Humble Decision Making." *Harvard Business Review* 67, no. 4 (1989): 122–26.

Evans, R. G. *Strained Mercy: The Economics of Canadian Healthcare.* Toronto: Butterworths, 1984.

Foster, J. "Hospitals in the Year 2000: A Scenario." *Frontiers of Health Services Management* 6, no. 2 (1989): 3–30.

Fox, W. L. "Vertical Integration Strategies: More Promising than Diversification." *Health Care Management Review* 14, no. 3 (1989): 49–56.

Friedman, E. "Marginal Missions and Missionary Margins." *Healthcare Forum Journal* 33, no. 1 (1990): 8–12.

Gardner, J. W. *On Leadership.* New York: The Free Press–Macmillan, 1990.

Goldsmith, J. "A Radical Prescription for Hospitals." *Harvard Business Review* 67, no. 3 (1989): 104–11.

Isenberg, D. J. "How Senior Managers Think." *Harvard Business Review* 62, no. 6 (1984): 80–90.

Jackall, R. "Moral Mazes: Bureaucracy and Managerial Work." *Harvard Business Review* 61, no. 5 (1983): 118–30.

Kaluzny, A. "Revitalizing Decision Making at the Middle Management Level." *Hospital & Health Services Administration* 34, no. 1 (1989): 39–51.

Kaluzny, A., and S. M. Shortell. "Creating and Managing the Future." In *Health Care Management: A Text in Organizational Theory and Behavior*, 2d. ed., 492–522. New York: Wiley, 1988.

Kanter, R. M. "The New Managerial Work." *Harvard Business Review* 67, no. 6 (1989): 85–92.

Kinzer, D. "Twelve Laws of Hospital Interaction." *Health Care Management Review* 15, no. 1 (1990): 47–60.

―――. "Where Is Hospital Leadership Coming From?" *Frontiers of Health Services Management* 3, no. 2 (1986): 3–26.

―――. "Why the Conservatives Gave Us Universal Health Care: A Parable." *Hospital & Health Services Administration* 34, no. 3 (1989): 299–310.

McCoy, B. H. "The Parable of the Sadhu." *Harvard Business Review* 61, no. 5 (1983): 103–8.

McLaughlin, C. P., and A. D. Kaluzny. "Total Quality Management in Health: Making It Work." *Health Care Management Review* 15, no. 3 (1990): 7–14.

Mullaney, A. D. "Downsizing: How One Hospital Responded to Decreasing Demand." *Health Care Management Review* 14, no. 3 (1989): 41–48.

Odiorne, G. S. *The Change Resisters.* Englewood Cliffs, NJ: Prentice-Hall, 1981.

O'Toole, J. *Vanguard Management.* Garden City, NY: Doubleday, 1985.

Ottensmeyer, D. J., and H. L. Smith. "Patterns of Medical Practice in an Era of Change." *Frontiers of Health Services Management* 3, no. 1 (1986): 3–29.

Peters, T., and N. Austin. *A Passion for Excellence.* New York: Random House, 1985, 263–414.

Quinn, J. B. "Managing Innovation: Controlled Chaos." *Harvard Business Review* 63, no. 3 (1985): 73–84.

Rohrer, J. E. "The Secret of Medical Management." *Health Care Management Review* 14, no. 3 (1989): 7–13.

Ross, A., S. J. Williams, and E. L. Schafer. *Ambulatory Care Management*, 2d. ed. Albany, NY: Delmar, 1991.

Rosenberg, M. L. "Patients and Hospitals." In *A Perspective on Patients*, 198–208. New York: Harcourt, Brace, and Jovanovich, 1981.

Schaef, A. W., and D. Fassel. *The Addictive Organization*. San Francisco: Harper & Row, 1988, 205–26.

Schroeder, L. "Cornucopia Management." *Administrative Radiology* (July 1990): 16–20.

Schwartz, F. N. "Management Women and the New Facts of Life." *Harvard Business Review* 67, no. 1 (1989): 65–76.

Scott, W. G., and D. K. Hart. *Organizational America*. Boston: Houghton Mifflin, 1979.

Scott, W. R. "Innovation in Medical Care Organizations: A Synthetic Review." *Medical Care Review* 47, no. 2 (1990): 165–92.

Shortell, S. M. *Effective Hospital-Physician Relationships*. Ann Arbor, MI: Health Administration Press, 1991.

———. "The Keys to Successful Diversification: Lessons from Leading Hospital Systems." *Hospital & Health Services Administration* 34, no. 4 (1989): 471–92.

———. "The Medical Staff of the Future." In *Health Services Management: Readings and Commentary*, 4th ed., edited by A. R. Kovner and D. Neuhauser, 316–44. Ann Arbor, MI: Health Administration Press, 1987.

Silas, C. J. "A Question of Scruples—Repairing Our Moral Compass." *Vital Speeches of the Day* (March 1989): 473–76.

Starr, P. *Social Transformation of American Medicine*. New York: Basic Books, 1982.

Umbdenstock, R., and W. Hageman. "The Five Critical Areas for Effective Governance of Not-For-Profit Hospitals." *Hospital & Health Services Administration* 35, no. 4 (1990): 481–92.

Zaleznik, A. "Real Work." *Harvard Business Review* 67, no. 1 (1989): 57–64.

INDEX

ABOUT THE AUTHOR

Austin Ross is Vice President and Executive Administrator of the Virginia Mason Medical Center in Seattle. Born in Milwaukee, Wisconsin, he attended the University of California at Berkeley, where he earned his bachelor's degree in business. After graduation, he served in the U.S. Army in the Korean War.

Upon completion of his duty with the Medical Services Corp, Ross returned to Berkeley and earned his M.P.H. degree. He took a residency in administration at the Virginia Mason Hospital in 1955 and has been with Virginia Mason since that time.

Also an active teacher, Ross has been a clinical professor at the University of Washington School of Public Health since 1977, and an adjunct instructor of health administration at Washington University School of Medicine since 1988. In addition, he is a member of the Association of University Programs in Health Administration.

Ross's professional activities include serving as Chairman of the American College of Healthcare Executives in 1984–85, as President of the Medical Group Management Association in 1976–77, and as President of the Association of Western Hospitals (Health Care Forum) in 1976–77. He has also served as a board member and committee member for these and other professional organizations. In addition, Ross has been a consultant for and served on special project committees for both the W. K. Kellogg Foundation and the Robert Wood Johnson Foundation.

Ross has been the recipient of numerous awards, including the 1989 Gold Medal Award for Distinguished Service from the American College of Healthcare Executives, the 1987 Executive Administrator of the Year Award from the American Group Practice Association, and the 1983 Harry J.

Harwick Award for Distinguished Service from the American College of Medical Group Administrators.

A regular contributor to the management literature, Ross's special interests lie in leadership, governance, and strategic planning issues. He has written on these topics for numerous journals and is the co-author, with Stephen J. Williams and Eldon L. Schafer, of *Ambulatory Care Management*, Second Edition, published in 1990 by Delmar Publishers.